# PANOS DOSSIER

Charlotte Watts

£6.95

UN
£2

D1584232

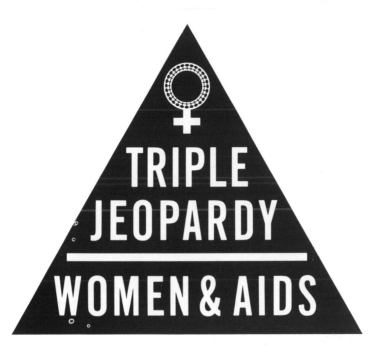

TRIPLE JEOPARDY

WOMEN & AIDS

## The Panos Institute
### Budapest — London — Paris — Washington

# ACKNOWLEDGEMENTS

Panos wishes to acknowledge the help given by many individuals and organisations across the world in compiling this dossier. Many of the writers credited in the text also gave much valuable background information not reproduced here. Many other individuals helped in a number of ways, including reviewing earlier drafts of this dossier. Space does not allow us to thank everyone by name, but we would like to include the following: Priscilla Alexander, Peri Batliwala, Aida Brako, Don Edwards, Dr Marie Thérèse Feuerstein, Sheila Gilchrist, Caroline Guinness, Dr Diane Gibb, Cathy Gilkes, Gill Gordon, Dr Anne Johnson, Naila Kabeer, Dr Andrea Kovacs, Dr Danielle Mercey, Dr Margaret Oxtoby, Dr Nancy Padian, Dr Martha Rogers, Dr Jane Rowley, Sunny Rumsey, Marie St Cyr, Dr Peter Selwyn, Jon Tinker, Nigel Twose, Ernesto de la Vega, Dr Eka Williams, Dr Debrework Zewdie.

Published by Panos Publications Ltd
9 White Lion Street  London N1 9PD, UK
British Library Cataloguing in Publication Data
Triple Jeopardy
1. Women. AIDS
I. Panos Institute
616.97920082
ISBN 1-870670-20-5

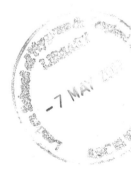

Extracts may be freely produced by the press or non-profit organisations, with or without acknowledgement. Panos would appreciate clippings of published material based on *Triple Jeopardy: Women and AIDS*. Funding for *Triple Jeopardy* was provided by the Norwegian Red Cross, Save the Children Fund (UK), Redd Barna (Save the Children Fund, Norway) and MISEREOR. The Panos AIDS Unit also receives financial support from the Swedish International Development Authority, the UK Overseas Development Administration and the Ford Foundation.

Any judgements expressed in this document should not be taken to represent the views of any funding agency. Signed articles do not necessarily reflect the views of Panos or any of its funding agencies.

An initial draft for this dossier was by Marty Radlett. It was researched and written by Judith Mariasy and Laura Thomas and coordinated by Judith Mariasy. Other writers are acknowledged where their contribution appears in the text. The dossier was edited by Olivia Bennett.

The Panos Institute is an information and policy studies institute, dedicated to working in partnership with others towards greater public understanding of sustainable development. Panos has offices in Budapest, London, Paris and Washington DC. The Panos AIDS and Development Information Unit supports research and publication on the extent and social impact of HIV/AIDS worldwide. The unit is directed by Martin Foreman.

For more information about Panos contact: Juliet Heller, The Panos Institute
Production: Sally O'Leary and Barbara Cheney
Picture research: Adrian Evans  Cover design: Viridian
Printed in Great Britain by The Southampton Book Company, Southampton

# CONTENTS

## THE GLOBAL PICTURE

HIV and AIDS — Means of transmission — The extent of the epidemic — Myths that miss the mark — Patterns of infection

## HOW ARE WOMEN AT RISK?

How risky is risky? — The mechanics of sexual transmission — Co-factors for sexual transmission — Non-sexual transmission — Who, me? Perceived versus actual risk

## A QUESTION OF CHOICE?

Sexual behaviour and choice — Negotiating safer sex — The power to choose — Cultural constraints on choice — The poverty factor

## HIV INFECTION, REPRODUCTION AND MOTHERHOOD

HIV disease in women — Does pregnancy affect an HIV-positive woman? — Mother-to-child transmission — To test or not to test? — Childbearing choice — Living with HIV

## HIV DISEASE IN INFANTS

Sources of infection — Detecting infant infection — Disease progression in children — Treatment for infected children — The ethics of experimental drugs for children

# PREFACE

In 1989, the Society for Women and AIDS in Africa (SWAA) first used the phrase "triple jeopardy" to describe the dangers women face as individuals, mothers and carers in the face of the AIDS pandemic. The founding of SWAA the previous year was part of a growing international awareness of the increasing threat of HIV to women and the importance of women-centred HIV prevention and care programmes. Almost 10 years into the epidemic, it was not before time.

This dossier, published to mark World AIDS Day 1990 which focuses on women and AIDS, is an important step forward in that process of awareness and action. Medical issues are clearly laid out alongside the social, economic and political constraints on women's behaviour and choices. The information is as vital for individuals as for AIDS service organisations and policy-makers worldwide.

AIDS is much more than a medical issue. It raises many of the fundamental questions of equity — between the sexes and between regions of the world — at the heart of the development debate. The stronger women's position in society, the greater their options for HIV prevention. This timely and important report from Panos tells us how and why in women's own words.

Dr Eka Williams
Secretary General
Society for Women and AIDS in Africa (SWAA)
September 1990

# AIDS: An issue for every woman

"In our communities whole families are dying. I watched my mother-in-law lose three sons — one who died of AIDS, my husband who was diagnosed with HIV-related illness after he died, and one who suspected that he had AIDS and died from a drug overdose. Two years after that she buried a daughter-in-law also from AIDS. A whole generation has been wiped out [1]."
*Sallie Perryman, herself HIV-positive, special assistant to the director, AIDS Institute, New York State Department of Health*

"The prospect of not being able to have children was — for me — at least as daunting as the possibility of a premature death. I needed the support of other women who had been through a similar process of saying good-bye to a future with children [2]."
*Amanda Heggs, a British woman living in Denmark, who is HIV-positive*

"The women tell us they see their husbands with the wives of men who have died of AIDS. And they ask, 'What can we do? If we say no, they'll say: pack up and go. But if we do, where do we go to?' They are dependent on the men and they have nowhere to go. What advice can you give these women [3]?"
*Miria Matembe, member of the Ugandan parliament and chairperson of Action for Development*

"Another time I took my son Johnny for an ear evaluation. I arrived at the hospital early...and was still there late in the afternoon when they asked me to leave because it was time to close the office. I started a big fuss. The nurse in charge didn't want to deal with my son out of fear of contamination. The doctor told me he was going to ask somebody else to do it and I refused. I wanted her to do it. I wanted her to learn that she couldn't be contaminated by doing that evaluation [4]."
*Maru Antuñano, Puerto Rican journalist. She and her son are HIV-positive*

"[The doctors] say there is something wrong in my blood because I slept with different men. Every night I pray that God will make my blood clean again so I can go home. I promise I won't return to prostitution again. I just want my mother; she will take care of me [5]."
*Selvi, 17-year-old prostitute with HIV detained for some years in Madras and released after a court case (see page 85)*

"There was a time when I used to sit on the London [underground train] and wonder what people would do if they knew I was HIV-positive. I felt totally alone. But now, when I think of how trendy it was to be bisexual in certain circles in the early 80s, of how many people have experimented with drugs, of the fact that 95% of gay [homosexual] men have slept with a woman at one point in their lives, then I no longer feel so alone. I don't sit on the tube and think, 'I am the only one', I sit on the tube and think, 'I wonder how many of you are positive?' [6]."
*Mary, a British woman in her thirties who is HIV-positive*

"Again and again I have to explain to an unsuspecting mother that her child may have a disease that she has never heard of and that I cannot cure....By the time that the child is admitted for the last time, I often know the mother well and the difficulties that she has faced because of the infection. But when the child dies I have no time to comfort the mother, because another baby has been admitted and the clinic is crowded. I am busy all the time, so I have no time to cry [7]."
*Dr Wendy Holmes, formerly government medical officer in a provincial hospital in Zimbabwe*

"A young woman of 27 came to us with AIDS. She had contracted it from her lover who was an injecting drug user, which she wasn't. She came to us during her second bout of pneumonia with a prescription she couldn't afford. She still — after three bouts of pneumonia — has not received any social security. This is the reality of the black community. I don't know whether they do it by zip code or by looking at your face. But I cannot understand why I have to go with her and appeal the fact that she's not eligible for social security. I don't know what more she has to prove after three bouts of pneumonia which have left her so thin she can hardly stand — maybe she has to die? Two other siblings are positive. One has already been into hospital two or three times....The other found out that he was positive when he was going into the army. His wife was already pregnant. Now everyone's hoping the baby's going to be all right [8]."
*Marie St Cyr, executive director of the Women's Action Resource Network in New York*

"There is no pattern emerging: there is no group that is more at risk than any other. We're in contact with teenagers to grandmothers of every class and ethnic group.Over three-quarters of the women who contact us have acquired the virus heterosexually [9]."
*Sheila Gilchrist, director of the UK-based support group Positively Women*

# CHAPTER 1

# THE GLOBAL PICTURE

Eight to ten million people are estimated to be infected with HIV — the virus which leads to AIDS — according to the World Health Organization (WHO). About one-third are women [10]. Overwhelmingly, they have contracted the virus through heterosexual intercourse, which globally is the major route for HIV transmission, accounting for about 60% of all infections by 1990. WHO expects that 75-80% of HIV infections will have resulted from heterosexual intercourse by the year 2000 [11].

In many industrialised countries, however, there remains the impression that HIV and AIDS only affect certain minority population groups such as homosexual men and injecting drug users and recipients of blood transfusions or blood products, particularly men with haemophilia. The true impact of HIV/AIDS on women is little recognised and rarely documented.

In those countries of the developing world where HIV has spread predominantly through heterosexual intercourse, there is greater awareness of the impact of HIV on women but often scant attention is paid to their specific needs. As women are at risk, so too are any future children they may have. Within a family, HIV often affects more than one person. Infection is commonly passed between sexual partners, and from mother to new-born infant. And in addition to

No risk in a kiss says a Spanish government cartoon.

## Means of transmission

HIV can be transmitted through blood and seminal or vaginal fluid. It can therefore pass from one person to another in three ways:
- via unprotected sexual intercourse (intercourse without a condom) with an infected person
- via infected blood — in transfusions, blood products and through the re-use of needles, syringes or other skin-piercing instruments

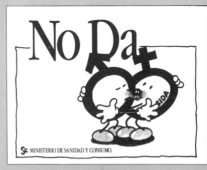

- from an infected mother to her baby — before, during or after birth

HIV is a virus which does not survive easily outside the body. There is no evidence that it has been transmitted in the everyday circumstances of home, school, the workplace, restaurants or any public place, or on toilet seats, by hugging, kissing or shaking hands, by sharing cups or cutlery, from coughing or from mosquito or other insect bites [45].

# HIV and AIDS

AIDS — Acquired Immune Deficiency Syndrome — is the term used to refer to the physical condition resulting from infection by HIV — the Human Immunodeficiency Virus. HIV is the generic term for two similar viruses known as HIV-1 and HIV-2, which are transmitted in the same ways (see box on previous page) and which both result in AIDS. HIV-1 has been detected worldwide; HIV-2 is most common in West Africa but has also been detected in North America, South America and Europe [41].

Being infected with HIV does not automatically mean that a person has AIDS or is ill. It does mean that a person can transmit HIV to someone else.

HIV gradually disables an important part of the body's immune system. Its main targets are cells in the blood called "T-helper cells", which HIV invades and eventually destroys. These cells normally help protect the body from attack by infection. As the immune system is progressively damaged, a person becomes increasingly vulnerable to a range of infections.

Because a variety of symptoms can occur in a person infected with HIV even prior to a diagnosis of AIDS, some experts now prefer to talk about "HIV infection and related disease" rather than HIV infection and AIDS. In mid-1990, WHO proposed a staging system of four parts to describe the patterns of ill health which result from HIV infection. The fourth stage corresponds to AIDS [42]. (See Chapter 4.)

The average time of progression from infection with HIV to the onset of AIDS (as defined by WHO and US Centers for Disease Control in 1987) — the incubation period — is approximately 10 years. Some people stay healthy for a much shorter period than this, but few develop AIDS within the first three years of infection [43]. Researchers estimate that others may be infected with HIV for up to 20 years before the onset of serious illness. People with HIV-2 seem to stay healthy longer than people with HIV-1 [44]. Once a person has developed AIDS, however, it seems to be almost invariably fatal.

It is not known exactly why some people stay healthy longer than others after contracting HIV. One reason is thought to be that HIV mutates frequently into slightly different forms, some of which appear to be more harmful and to replicate more quickly than others. Another possibility is that people who already have a weak immune system, as the result of other infections such as malaria, tuberculosis or malnutrition, may succumb more quickly to the effects of HIV infection.

During this long period without symptoms, the way HIV infection can be detected is by testing a person's blood. The most common test involves checking a blood sample for the presence of HIV antibodies. Antibodies are defence compounds produced by the body in response to an invading organism — such as a virus. The presence of antibodies in a person's blood shows that they have been exposed to that virus. In the case of HIV, this will give rise to an HIV-positive test result.

coping with their own infection and illness, women usually find themselves responsible for caring for the entire household. It is not surprising that in Zambia AIDS is known as "the family disease".

## THE EXTENT OF THE EPIDEMIC

By September 1990, WHO had reported 283,010 cases of AIDS worldwide. Of these, 50% were in the United States, and 25%, 14% and 9% in sub-Saharan Africa, Europe, and Latin America and the Caribbean respectively. The rest of the world accounted for less than

## HIV infection and AIDS — global estimates for 1990

| | CUMULATIVE TOTAL AIDS CASES | TOTAL HIV-POSITIVE | TOTAL WOMEN* HIV-POSITIVE | PERCENTAGE WOMEN* HIV-POSITIVE |
|---|---|---|---|---|
| NORTH AMERICA | 175,000 | 1,000,000 | 100,000 | 0.14 |
| LATIN AMERICA (includes the Caribbean) | 75,000 | 1,000,000 | 200,000 | 0.2 |
| EUROPE | 50,000 | <500,000 | 60,000 | 0.03 |
| AFRICA | >500,000 | >5,000,000 | >2,500,000 | 2.5 |
| ASIA | >1,000 | 500,000 | 200,000 | 0.03 |
| OCEANIA | <1,000 | 30,000 | 3,000 | 0.06 |

\* Women aged 15-49
> more than
< less than

Source: World Health Organization Global Programme on AIDS, September 1990

3% of cases. However, these figures may be inaccurate because in many countries, particularly in the developing world, reporting of cases is often delayed and incomplete. A more accurate estimate of AIDS cases, calculated by WHO to take under-reporting into account, is given in the box above.

Even the figures for AIDS cases in the above table do not give an accurate picture of the current state of the epidemic. Because the average incubation period is approximately 10 years, reported numbers of AIDS cases only indicate how many people were infected at an uncertain point in the past; they do not reveal how many people have HIV today.

A more accurate indication of levels of infection comes from the results of blood tests which detect exposure to HIV among selected groups of the population; these may be patients attending sexually transmitted disease (STD) clinics, hospital outpatients, blood donors, male and female prostitutes, injecting drug users and pregnant women or new-born babies (who carry their mothers' antibodies to HIV for several months whether or not they are infected themselves). The process of testing large groups of people for the epidemiological purpose of mapping the path of HIV is known as screening; screening of similar population groups over time gives an indication of the developing course of the epidemic.

Such data must nevertheless be interpreted cautiously since it is not always possible to make generalisations from information which relates to particular individuals. HIV infection is seldom distributed

# Myths that miss the mark

Blood survey results clearly lay to rest the myth that HIV and AIDS only affect "high-risk groups", often assumed to be male. Women everywhere, especially young women, and children are increasingly at risk.

### Myth 1: Women don't get HIV/AIDS

* AIDS is now the leading cause of death for women aged 20-40 in major cities in the Americas, Western Europe, and sub-Saharan Africa. Between 1989 and 1992 the number of women infected with HIV in sub-Saharan Africa is expected to increase by more than 60% and the number of infected children to double [46].
* In West and Central African countries, approximately equal numbers of men and women have developed AIDS, although some studies show more infected women in some cities [47]. (Differences in rates of infection amongst men and women must be interpreted cautiously. The circumstances in which population groups are selected for testing may bias positive results towards women or towards men.)
* In the United States — where HIV has so far spread mainly among gay (homosexual) men and injecting drug users — women now account for just over 10% of AIDS cases. In the year ending July 1990, at least 34% of new AIDS cases among US women and 3% of new AIDS cases among US men resulted from heterosexual intercourse [48]. In New York, the worst affected state, accounting for almost a quarter of all AIDS cases in the country, 17.3% of cases reported in 1989 were among women [49].
* In Europe one in six people diagnosed with AIDS in the year ending April 1990 were women [50].

### Myth 2: Teenagers don't get HIV/AIDS

* At least half of all people infected with HIV worldwide are under the age of 25. About one-fifth of all people who have developed AIDS to date are in their twenties [51]. Because of the slow rate of progression from HIV infection to AIDS, many must have been infected in their teens.
* The ratio of male to female cases of HIV is dramatically different in some countries among young men and women compared with older adults. One Zairean study showed women aged between 15 and 30 to be four times more likely to have HIV than men in the same age group [52]. Other STDs show a similar bias towards young women. For example, in the United Kingdom in 1987, women accounted for 60% of cases of gonorrhoea reported in people under the age of 20. The male to female ratio was reversed in people above the age of 20 [53].
* A 1990 US study of over a million teenage army applicants found that levels of infection among young men and women were roughly equal, although the country has reported nearly nine times as many AIDS cases among men as among women. Because risk data were not collected, the contribution of injecting drug use, heterosexual or homosexual sex and social and economic influences to HIV infection levels was unclear. The researchers say that "the most likely reason for the higher prevalences among 17- and 18-year-old [women] is that they are more likely to have older, infected sexual partners than are males [54]".

**Myth 3: Infants don't get HIV/AIDS**
- It is estimated that during the 1980s over 550,000 infants worldwide were born HIV-positive; approximately 90% of these were in sub-Saharan Africa [55]. Where levels of HIV infection in women are high and women have higher levels of fertility, the opportunities for mother-to-child transmission of HIV are much greater [56].
- AIDS is a sizeable new risk of death for young children in areas of the world where child survival is already threatened. In some Central African studies between 10% and 20% of pregnant women are infected. In a country where 100 children in every 1,000 die before the age of five (a situation common in many developing countries), this level of infection would cause child deaths to increase from 100 per 1,000 to between 118 and 136 per 1,000 [57]. "The advances of child-survival programmes of the past 20 years may already be reversed," according to WHO experts [58]. By comparison, in most industrial countries fewer than 20 children per 1,000 die from all causes.
- In the United States, AIDS is already the ninth leading cause of death among one- to four-year-olds [59]. Almost 2,500 children had been diagnosed with AIDS by July 1990 [60].

evenly throughout a country's population. Major cities just a few kilometres apart can report dramatically different levels of infection. For example, up to 50% of injecting drug users tested in Edinburgh, United Kingdom, are infected. Seventy kilometres away in Glasgow, the estimated level of infection in a similar group has never been more than 6% [12]. In the Rakai district of Uganda, levels of HIV infection vary widely, from a low of 1.2% in some areas to 52.8% in others [13].

In 1985, about half of the global total of HIV infections were estimated to be in the developing world. By 1990, on the basis of new and improved blood survey data, this proportion had risen to two-thirds of the estimated 8-10 million people infected. Further rises to as high as 75-80% and 80-90% are projected by the year 2000 and 2010 respectively [14]. In mid-1990 Dr Michael Merson, newly appointed director of WHO's Global Programme on AIDS, stated that the main message of these figures was that "the toll of HIV infection around the globe is worsening rapidly, especially in developing countries". He added that "if HIV prevalence over the next couple of years increases markedly in Asia and Latin America, and continues to expand in sub-Saharan Africa, then our projections — which are considered conservative — will need to be revised even further upward [15]".

Using the information from the improved blood surveys reported in 1990, WHO constructed an epidemiologically based "AIDS projection model" to estimate the current levels of HIV infection in women and children around the world and to make short-term predictions of future levels. The model estimated that by the end of 1992, sub-Saharan Africa would see a total of 600,000 cases of AIDS in women and a similar number in children. Four million women and

*The toll of HIV infection around the globe is worsening rapidly, especially in developing countries*

one million children would have been infected with the virus. This would likely represent about 90% of all cases of HIV infection in women and children worldwide [16].

## PATTERNS OF INFECTION

Early in the epidemic, WHO identified regions by predominant modes of transmission.

- North America, Western Europe, Australia and New Zealand, where the overwhelming majority of people with HIV were men infected through homosexual transmission or men and women infected by sharing needles for drug use, were denoted pattern I.
- Sub-Saharan Africa, where the overwhelming majority of those with HIV were infected heterosexually, and where in consequence HIV infection among children was relatively high, was pattern II.
- The Middle East, Asia and Eastern Europe, where extensive spread of HIV began in the mid to late 1980s via blood transfusion and sexual transmission, were pattern III.
- Latin America and the Caribbean were originally deemed to be pattern I areas, but the increasing number of women infected heterosexually caused WHO to redesignate the region pattern I/II.

Within this broad classification, patterns of infection within a region vary from country to country. Furthermore, they are not static. In the United Kingdom, for example, although the majority of people who are HIV-positive are gay (homosexual) men and injecting drug users, people who acquire HIV through heterosexual intercourse make up a rising percentage of those affected[17]. In the United States, the 1980s public perception of people with AIDS as middle-class, white, homosexual men has been revised in the 1990s as disproportionate levels of infection among black and Latino men and women in underprivileged communities became apparent. From very few cases of infection in the mid-1980s, Thailand now reports accelerating HIV spread. Infection is spreading in three ways: through shared needles, and unprotected homosexual and heterosexual sex. Only in sub-Saharan Africa has the pattern of transmission — predominantly unprotected heterosexual intercourse — remained constant across the region and over a period of years.

### Women, heterosexual spread and drug use

Among industrialised countries, the United States has reported the largest number of AIDS cases in women and children: 13,395 and 2,464 respectively at the end of July 1990 [18]. These cases, however, only represent the tip of the iceberg.

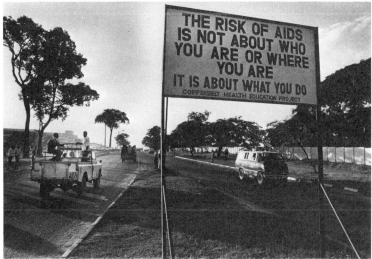

Highway headlines: messages that can't be missed in Zambia tell drivers they cannot avoid HIV by assuming it is someone else's problem. Risks are firmly attached to activities and not to particular groups of people.
*Ron Giling/Panos Pictures*

Estimates from 24 US states suggest that three out of every 2,000 childbearing women nationwide are HIV-positive. Even this national average can be misleading. Some US inner cities have much higher rates of infection and some women face more risks than others. In the six states in this study with data on mothers' race, levels of HIV infection were 5 to 15 times higher among black women than among white women [19]. The identification of high levels of infection among black and Latino communities in this and other US studies is an indication of an underlying factor which helps the virus to spread in many parts of the world — disadvantage and poverty.

A major factor in this spread through inner-city communities is injecting drug use, reflecting "the frustration and anger of marginalized and impoverished populations seeking escape through mood-altering drugs," according to Don Edwards, former executive director of the US National Minority AIDS Council [20]. Injecting drug use in itself accounted for almost half of all female US AIDS cases in the year ending July 1990. In the same period over one-third of female AIDS cases resulted from heterosexual sex [21]. Black and Latina women are over-represented in these figures but the risk is not exclusive to poor urban communities [22].

In Europe, particularly in Switzerland, Italy, France and Spain, HIV has spread rapidly among injecting drug users and their sexual *The impact* partners. More than half of the 1,729 people who tested HIV-positive *of HIV is* in Scotland by the end of 1989 were injecting drug users. Many have *magnified* acknowledged their injecting risk but do not yet realise the extent to *by poverty* which unprotected sexual intercourse puts partners at risk, say *and under-* counsellors. In one city, Edinburgh, one in a 100 men between the *development* ages of 15 and 44 are estimated to be infected [23] and some researchers say heterosexual sex is now a more common means of transmission than needle sharing [24].

The number of women infected by unprotected heterosexual sex may even be slightly underestimated by those countries which use a hierarchical system to classify risk factors for AIDS. In the United States and the United Kingdom, for example, a drug-using woman with AIDS is classified according to her injecting risk rather than because she has sex with a drug-using partner, even though the latter may have been her source of infection.

## Bisexual men and their women partners

Some men have sexual relations both with women and other men. Many of these men marry and do not identify themselves as bisexual or homosexual. Some studies suggest that men who do not acknowledge their bisexual behaviour are less likely to use condoms with their female partners than with their male partners [25].

The first appearance of AIDS in Latin America and the Caribbean was in men who had contracted the virus through unprotected homosexual sex. But because a significant number of men in the region have intercourse with both sexes [26], infection has spread increasingly to women. By mid-1990, 20% of HIV infections in South America were estimated to be in women [27].

In Brazil, which has reported the greatest number of AIDS cases in Latin America, unprotected bisexual sex has had a greater influence on heterosexual spread than injecting drug use — which is generally confined to specific areas, such as Rio de Janeiro and São Paulo [28]. Similar trends are emerging in other Latin American countries. In Mexico, the ratio of male to female infection was 7:1 in December 1989. The following April it stood at 5:1 [29]. In late 1989, Honduras reported a male to female ratio of infection of 1.3:1. In April that year, 13.7% of the country's AIDS cases occurred among homosexual men and 13.3% in bisexual men. The "truly surprising fact" say researchers, is that 65.8% of the cases have occurred among heterosexuals — nearly half of them women. Seven per cent were female prostitutes, "but the remainder...most likely represent women infected by bisexual men" [30]. Some countries in the Caribbean show the same trend. In 1983, many Trinidadians believed HIV was exclusively confined to homosexual and bisexual men. During 1989, however, figures showed that 43% of AIDS cases occurred among heterosexuals. Many must have been infected several years earlier. The male to female ratio of infection in Trinidad fell from 19:1 in

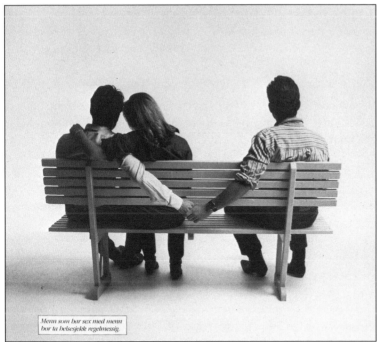

Menn som har sex med menn bor ta helsesjekk regelmessig.

"Men who have sex with men should have regular health checks," advises a Norwegian poster. Studies show that many men who do not acknowledge their bisexuality are less likely to use condoms — particularly with their female partners.
*Oslo helseråd*

1984 to 3:1 in 1989 [31].

The phenomenon of women at risk of infection from unprotected sex with a bisexual partner who may have been exposed to HIV is not unique to Latin America and the Carribean. In the United Kingdom, for example, according to a 1990 report, over 10% of homosexual men said they had had sex with a female partner within the previous year [32].

## Heterosexual spread

In Central, Eastern and Southern Africa and in some parts of the Caribbean, men and women have been infected with HIV in roughly equal numbers, primarily through heterosexual sex, since the beginning of the epidemic. In sub-Saharan Africa, one in 40 adult men and women are estimated to be HIV-positive [33], but the picture is far from uniform across the region. Some countries are particularly badly affected, while others are relatively untouched.

The reasons for such widespread infection in sub-Saharan Africa, and the implications for women, are examined in later chapters of this dossier. The impact of HIV in developing countries is magnified by poverty and underdevelopment, which limit available health programmes and threaten community stability. In some of the most heavily affected countries in Africa, inadequate access to basic health services has meant that many people are not effectively treated for sexually transmitted diseases — which in themselves appear to be significant co-factors in HIV transmission (see Chapter 2).

## An open door

A few years ago it seemed that AIDS was knocking on the door of Asia. That door is now wide open. In mid-1990, WHO reported that the total number of people with HIV in Asia had risen from virtually nil two years previously to an estimated total of at least 500,000 — a much more rapid increase than had been predicted. WHO warned that estimates of HIV infections in Asia by the year 2000 — between 1.0 and 1.5 million — might have to be revised dramatically upwards if current trends continued [34].

In Thailand in the mid-1980s, cases of HIV infection were restricted to the extensive networks of homosexual prostitutes catering for foreign visitors. By 1988, HIV was spreading rapidly within a second population: Thailand's estimated 100,000 injecting drug users [35]. Testing among some groups of Thai drug users found nearly half were HIV-positive by mid-1990, according to WHO [36]. Heterosexual transmission of HIV is emerging as a significant problem. Poorly paid women in the Thai sex industry are particularly affected. At the end of 1989, the average rates of HIV infection among different groups of sex workers, many of whom cater for international sex tourists, ranged from nearly 2% to almost 7% — double the figures recorded six months earlier. The sex ratio of people with HIV rose from one woman for every 17 men in 1986 to one woman for every five men in 1990 [37].

Reports from India show that HIV is making rapid inroads. Over 100,000 blood donations tested in Bombay in 1989 revealed that 0.14% of those who gave blood voluntarily were HIV-positive. Among donors who sell blood, generally as a means of livelihood, 2.4% tested positive [38]. Meanwhile, tests between September 1986 and January 1990 showed that 6.2% of nearly 2,000 women working in the "red light" areas of Bombay tested positive. Initially few women were infected, but among those tested in the six-month period up to January 1990, almost one-quarter were HIV-positive [39].

Other countries are also increasingly affected, although figures on the impact on women are not always available. Infection in Sri Lanka and Indonesia — still uncommon — is associated with homosexual transmission, while infection resulting from sharing needles for drug use has been detected in China, India and Malaysia.

## A major challenge

Although the exact level of HIV infection among women worldwide is not known, evidence exists to show that millions are already HIV-positive, and that millions more are likely to become infected before the end of the century. In the words of WHO, HIV infection in women is set to become "one of the major challenges to public health, health care and social support systems worldwide" [40].

HIV and AIDS are a potential threat to women all over the world. This dossier contains examples, information and testimony from many countries but has necessarily concentrated on two areas: Africa, where HIV infection among women is believed to be most widespread; and the United States, which reports the greatest number of affected women in the industrialised world and where resources have allowed most research on the epidemic.

Wherever it strikes, the epidemic of HIV/AIDS has an impact far beyond that of individual illness and early death. The Human Immunodeficiency Virus affects every aspect of women's lives, whether or not they themselves are infected. Some of these aspects are examined in the following chapters.

# CHAPTER 2

# HOW ARE WOMEN AT RISK?

W omen and men are at risk of HIV infection through unprotected sexual intercourse and infected blood. As no vaccine or effective treatment for the disease yet exists, the only way people can protect themselves and each other from HIV infection is to avoid behaviour known to be risky.

This chapter looks at the mechanics of HIV infection and the risks to women, while Chapter 3 explores why responses to those risks, including the options of chastity, faithful partnerships or safer sex, are difficult or impossible for many to sustain. Whenever behaviour change is hampered — because of inadequate information, the constraints of poverty or powerlessness — women will be unable to protect themselves, and any future children.

## HOW RISKY IS RISKY?

Estimates of the probability of becoming infected with HIV are precarious for several reasons. Some infected people are more efficient transmitters of HIV than others, and some people may be more susceptible to infection. "Some partners have not become infected after literally thousands of [sexual] contacts. Others were infected after one," warns Dr Nancy Padian at the University of California at Berkeley, in the United States [1]. Some women whose partners are HIV-positive have had regular sex over several years without contracting HIV, even when they have not practised safer sex consistently [2].

In addition, transmission efficiency may vary according to the stage of the illness. Individuals may be particularly infectious just after becoming infected themselves and when they develop symptoms. However, because most people with HIV are currently not sick, most transmission occurs from those without symptoms.

Much of the information about heterosexual transmission of HIV comes from studies which compare men and women who have remained HIV-negative with those who have become positive during a sexual relationship with an HIV-positive partner. These studies have tried to assess why some people acquire the virus and others do not. They examine the risks associated with unprotected sexual intercourse as well as the influence of additional "co-factors" such as sexually transmitted diseases (STDs) — which increase both vulnerability to acquiring the virus and the likelihood that an infected person will transmit the virus.

*Men appear to pass on HIV more efficiently than women during unprotected vaginal intercourse*

Many studies find no consistent relationship between the number of times a couple have sexual intercourse and the likelihood of infection. Although frequency of sexual intercourse is likely to have some influence, researchers now think it is fairly meaningless to try to estimate a consistent risk per sexual encounter. Instead, because of the level of inconsistency they suggest the notion of variable risk [3]. In short, anyone who takes a risk cannot know the degree of risk involved.

## THE MECHANICS OF SEXUAL TRANSMISSION

Within this framework of variability there are degrees of certainty about the actual mechanics of HIV transmission.

HIV is carried in seminal and vaginal fluids and in cervical secretions as well as in blood. Any exchange of fluids during intercourse can result in transmission of the virus across the porous membranes of the vagina, penis or anal canal into the blood stream. The fact that seminal fluid transmits the virus is confirmed by studies of artificial insemination (AI). Women have even been infected by a single exposure to infected semen during AI [4].

### Unprotected vaginal intercourse

Where HIV is spread heterosexually, unprotected vaginal intercourse — intercourse without a condom — is the major risk. Several major studies in Europe and the United States, in which detailed sexual histories of partners were taken, show that almost 80% of women infected sexually reported unprotected vaginal intercourse as their only risk activity [5].

Men appear to pass on HIV more efficiently than women during unprotected vaginal intercourse, making women more likely to be infected by men than men to be infected by women, twice as likely say some researchers [6]. This does not mean men are not at risk. One study reports that several men have been infected after a single sexual encounter with an HIV-positive woman [7]. European and US studies suggest that on average, between 10 and 30% of women in steady relationships with HIV-positive men become infected, whereas some 5 to 15% of men are infected by their female partners [8].

This parallels figures which show that some other STDs, such as gonorrhoea, are more easily transmitted from men to women. The chances of male-to-female transmission of gonorrhoea are thought to be around 50-80% after a single exposure, and female-to-male around 20-25% [9].

Some researchers suggest that there is an as yet unconfirmed additional risk of infection for men, but not for women, from sex during menstruation, since HIV is carried in the blood as well as in genital secretions [10].

## Unprotected anal intercourse

Although often associated with sex between men, heterosexual couples may practise anal sex as a form of birth control, to preserve virginity, or for pleasure. Anal intercourse is more risky for women than unprotected vaginal intercourse — doubly so, according to some researchers [11].

## Oral sex

HIV infection through unprotected oral sex with a man or a woman is theoretically possible since seminal and vaginal fluids both carry the virus and minute cuts or sores in the mouth may provide an entry point for HIV.

It is considered to be substantially less risky than unprotected anal or vaginal sex but there are a few documented cases of HIV infection where oral sex, both between women [12] and between women and men, has been suggested but not confirmed as the means of transmission [13]. Condoms or dental dams (thin latex squares placed over a woman's genital area) can be used as protection. Information from users of dental dams is scarce but their efficacy against potential infection  and their practicality has been questioned by some [14].

## CO-FACTORS FOR SEXUAL TRANSMISSION

Variations in sexual practice or in how infectious a partner is, and thus how easily the virus is transmitted, are not the whole story. Other "co-factors" can increase the risk of HIV transmission.

## Sexually transmitted diseases

Research has confirmed that STDs such as chancroid, syphilis and genital herpes, sometimes collectively known as genital ulcer disease (GUD), are associated with increased rates of HIV transmission, independent of the risk associated with multiple partners. The genital ulcers caused by these infections provide an open door for HIV to pass from one sexual partner to another. A woman is more likely to be infected by an HIV-positive man who who has GUD than by one without it [15], and if she has GUD she is also more likely to pass on infection [16]. Treating a person for GUD may therefore significantly reduce the likelihood of him or her transmitting or becoming infected with HIV.

*Several STDs are linked to increased rates of HIV infection*

STDs which do not cause ulcers are also implicated [17]. Some studies show that women who become infected with HIV are more likely to have had infections which do not cause ulcers, such as cervical infections, gonorrhoea or chlamydial infection which can cause urethritis. Information about STDs which do not cause ulcers or which do cause painless sores is particularly important to women. A sore or discharge is more likely to be noticed in a man, whereas internal sores or inflammation often pass undetected in a woman, and inflammation alone can increase the risk of HIV transmission. Many STDs are relatively free of symptoms in women unless serious complications, such as pelvic inflammatory disease, result. Mild symptoms, such as lower abdominal pain, are sometimes simply regarded as "a woman's lot".

Although it can be transmitted by non-sexual means, HIV infection is primarily a sexually transmitted disease. When viewed in this way, AIDS becomes the latest manifestation of an enduring problem: that of high and rising rates of STDs.

More than 20 different diseases are spread by sexual contact, according to the World Health Organization (WHO), with an estimated 125 million cases of infection worldwide every year. Although infection levels are similar in both women and men, women and infants bear the brunt of the serious complications which often follow a bout of disease. In some areas of some developing countries congenital syphilis, for example, causes up to 25% of stillbirths and deaths in infants under one month. In the United States, syphilis cases increased by more than 50% between 1985 and 1989. Infertility, some pregnancy complications, and genital and anal cancers are often associated with STDs.

In industrialised countries, chlamydial infection and viral infections such as genital warts and genital herpes are increasingly common. Until recently, the most commonly identified STDs in many developing countries were the bacterial infections such as chancroid, syphilis and gonorrhoea. However, chlamydial and viral infections have started to be reported [18].

## Circumcision

There is currently no evidence linking female circumcision as a risk factor to HIV infection. The Society for Women and AIDS in Africa

*HIV infection through contaminated blood transfusions hits women disproportionately* (SWAA) reports that "in areas where this practice is still carried out the prevalence of HIV is low [19]". This could reflect the fact that HIV was introduced relatively recently into these areas or it could reflect traditional restrictions on the number of sexual partners in the societies concerned. However, any sex which involves bleeding increases the risk of HIV infection and some forms of female genital excision, and particularly infibulation, can lead to extensive bleeding during initial intercourse.

There is some evidence that uncircumcised men are more likely than circumcised men to contract and transmit HIV and other STDs [20]. Researchers suspect that the increased risk from being uncircumcised may stem from the fact that the foreskin traps vaginal fluid, provides a larger surface area for uptake of the virus and may be more susceptible to microscopic tears during sexual intercourse. In addition, minor inflammatory conditions are more common in uncircumcised men.

## Contraception

Sexually active women who do not wish to conceive want safe and reliable contraception. The condom is currently the contraceptive which offers the most reliable protection against HIV.

But millions of women use other forms of contraception. Does their choice of method have any bearing on their risk of contracting HIV? Information from early studies raised the possibility that the use of oral contraceptives might facilitate the transmission of HIV since they can be associated with cervical inflammation and bleeding [21]. This suggestion, however, remains controversial and is not supported by other evidence. Intra-uterine devices (IUDs) are known to increase the risk of pelvic inflammation and infections and despite the absence of detailed research, WHO recommends that they should not be used by women at risk from STDs, including HIV, or by women who are HIV-positive [22].

## NON-SEXUAL TRANSMISSION

HIV infection through contaminated blood transfusions hits women disproportionately, particularly women in the poorest communities of developing countries. Childbirth is the trigger. In Uganda, as many as three-quarters of all adult blood transfusions in 1988 were given to women, most of whom faced complications such as anaemia or severe bleeding in childbirth [23]. In 1990 WHO estimated that approximately 10% of AIDS cases in sub-Saharan Africa by that time had resulted from transfusions with infected blood [24]. Major improvements have been made since the risks became known and where the risk is *Even those* greatest, most blood is screened. Continent-wide this is estimated to *who know* amount to about 60% of blood used. Blood supplies are also protected *about the need* by advising those who may be particularly at risk for HIV infection *for safer sex* not to donate blood. In the Eastern Mediterranean and Asia not all *admit to not* countries routinely screen all blood, particularly where HIV infection *always* levels are low [25]. *practising it*

Many women are concerned about the risks they face from contaminated blood. "We women have to expose ourselves to so many more hospital procedures than men do — even when sterilisation is concerned, nine times out of ten it is the women who go through with it. Why?" asks Veena, an Indian woman. "What options do I have where hospitals are concerned? What if I have to have a blood transfusion for instance, or even a simple injection [26]?"

Contaminated blood also presents a risk for women using unsterilised needles and syringes, whether for medical reasons or through sharing drug users' equipment, known as "works". In most countries, more men than women have been infected through injecting drug use, but there is the accompanying risk of heterosexual transmission for the woman partner. And sharing "works" remains a major route of infection among women in the United States and Europe.

## WHO, ME? PERCEIVED VERSUS ACTUAL RISK

Knowing the odds for HIV transmission is important for attempts to predict the way the virus is likely to spread in a particular population. But how useful are statistical calculations for an individual?

The idea of risk is one of the most difficult concepts in health education. A person's own idea of his or her risk of HIV infection, like other threats to life or health, often bears little relation to actual risk. Even those who know all the facts about HIV and the need for safer sex sometimes admit to not always practising it themselves. As Heather Downs a volunteer on the women's group of the UK organisation, the Terrence Higgins Trust, points out: "Many women working in AIDS service organisations or in other areas which lead them to deal with AIDS health education find it difficult to connect the information they do have to their own lives, for example, in terms of negotiating safer sex with a new partner [27]." Rational intentions do not always materialise.

AIDS prevention programmes which advise women to insist on condom use or "Just Say No" campaigns do not recognize the realities

***Knowledge about HIV risk reduction is often used selectively*** of many people's lives. "Public health professionals often mistakenly assume that everyone goes through a rational decision-making process based on middle-class values when considering condom use; they do not look at the social costs to women of negotiating condom use — costs that vary across socioeconomic and ethnic groups," says US anthropologist Dr Dooley Worth [28].

The less bargaining power a woman has, the harder it is to avoid taking risks. Some women fear that if they insist upon condom use or even ask their partner to use a condom, they will endanger their relationship, perhaps even lose their partner. And in losing their partner they may lose a relationship which confers status, emotional and perhaps financial support. Those women with dependent children are especially vulnerable.

Knowledge about HIV risk reduction is often used selectively. For example, a woman working as a prostitute may insist on condom use with a client but not with a partner [29]. Several factors underlie this: some say it is easier for a woman to insist on condom use in a business setting where she has authority — an authority which may be lost in a personal setting. Equally important according to AIDS educators is the desire of prostitutes to "distinguish between 'work' and 'intimate' sex by not using condoms with their primary partner" [30]. Distinctions between "kinds" of sexual activity are not confined to sex workers. Many people who would not use condoms with their regular partner, would do so for a casual encounter. "When you are happy with someone you think 'I really want to be with this person' and the worry about picking up something from them is not so strong," said a young British woman interviewed about her own risk behaviour [31]. Studies have shown repeatedly that even people who begin by insisting on safer sex find this decision difficult to sustain [32]. For most people, sex with someone they know and love feels safer — but may not be. Perceived and actual risks do not always coincide. And for those who do get infected with HIV, analysis of the likelihood of infection is academic.

# CHAPTER 3

# A QUESTION OF CHOICE?

## SEXUAL BEHAVIOUR AND CHOICE

Men and women have the same options to protect themselves against HIV: chastity, faithful relationships, or non-penetrative or condom-protected sex. Both sexes suffer from complacency about or denial of the risks of HIV infection. But even those who recognise the risks cannot always translate this awareness into action. The AIDS pandemic has cast a spotlight on weaknesses in health and information services around the world. Many of these deficiencies affect women disproportionately. Furthermore, many of the cultural constraints on sexual decision-making particularly affect women and some behavioural scientists question whether there has been any serious attempt to look at the AIDS pandemic as a social phenomenon. "Social scientists are seen as ancilliary to medical researchers in a way that underestimates the importance of the science of sustained behaviour change," says Tanzanian researcher Dr Eustace Muhondwa [1].

*There has never been a society in which the patterns of sexual behaviour were restricted solely to monogamy or chastity*

"If we are to tackle the problem of HIV infection and AIDS, it is essential that we study not only the virus itself but all cultural practices which might contribute to its spread," says Nigerian researcher, Dr A. Nasidi [2]. With no immediate prospect of a widely-available vaccine or cure for HIV, the key to controlling the AIDS epidemic lies in sexual behaviour and its modification. But human behaviour is rooted in the social and economic facts of individual lives. At the beginning of the 1990s women's choices, particularly about sexual behaviour, are often subject to powerful and far-reaching constraints. As awareness of the spread of the virus grows, the critical limitations on the power of many women in their personal relationships are increasingly highlighted.

## Chastity

"There has never been a society in which the patterns of sexual behaviour were restricted solely to monogamy or chastity," says Professor June Osborne, of the US National AIDS Commission [3].

Every society has its culturally acceptable standards of sexual behaviour, such as when women and men may participate in sexual activity. In many cultures this is only sanctioned for women after marriage; for men it is more common to see sexual activity as

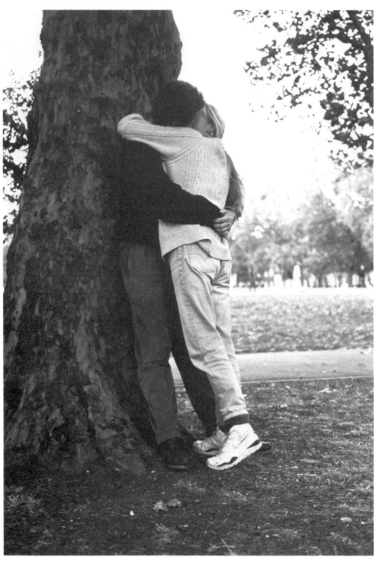

acceptable while they are single. Because of women's child-bearing potential, and their often lower economic and social status, the "rules" for their sexual behaviour have generally been stricter than those for men. But social norms and the reality of people's lives seldom coincide and evidence abounds of the gap between the two. Nevertheless, cultural expectations continue to exert powerful constraints over people's sexual behaviour and in many societies pre-marital chastity is the desired norm.

In the majority of industrialised countries, the age of menarche (first menstruation) is dropping because of improvements in health and nutrition. At the same time, increased education and social mobility mean that many women marry or form permanent relationships later in life. Thus the period between sexual maturity and the establishment of long-term partnerships is lengthening. In the United States, for example, at the end of the eighteenth century the age of menarche was 14 and the average age of marriage for women was 18; today first menstruation occurs between 12 and 13 years while women marry on average at age 23-24 [4]. Some 70% of US adolescents report having engaged in sexual intercourse by age 19, and 17% of males and 6% of females aged 16-19 report at least one homosexual experience [5]. The most common age of first intercourse for women in France, the Netherlands and the United Kingdom is about 18. Statistics on teenage pregnancy show that much of this sex is unprotected [6].

In developing countries, little research has been done on the sexual behaviour of adolescents. In many parts of the world adolescence may be very short, particularly where women are likely to enter partnerships and become mothers during their teenage years.

Clearly, throughout the world, whatever the prevailing social norm, many young unmarried people do engage in sexual activity, some at very young ages and many with a high degree of ignorance about how to avoid unwanted pregnancy or sexually transmitted diseases, including HIV infection. Safer sex or no sex — the choice is much easier to make if it is based on accurate and accessible information. AIDS educators say there is a great need to reach young people early, before they become sexually active. Successful approaches to sex education — many of which rely on harnessing the power of peer pressure — are described in Chapter 7.

## Partnerships

Marriages or partnerships implying patterns of sexual fidelity provide a norm of social organisation in most regions of the world. Many governments and some non-governmental organisations, particularly those affiliated with religious groups, are making fidelity messages a cornerstone of their AIDS prevention policies, especially where condoms are in short supply or are opposed on religious grounds. Yet mutual and permanent sexual fidelity requires joint commitment. Infidelity has proved to be a big issue in HIV prevention and education.

In cultures where serial monogamy is common — where people have a series of long-term relationships and are mutually faithful within each one — no couple, unless they are both virgins, can be sure

*Infidelity has proved to be a big issue in HIV prevention and education*

that they or any previous partners have never been at risk sexually, given that the incubation period for HIV averages 10 years. In addition, evidence confirms what many recognise as reality: that men and women will lie in order to have sex. A research project in the United States revealed that about one-third of nearly 200 male college students aged 18-25 admitted they had lied to a woman about their sexual and drug-using history in order to have sex, compared to 10% of the same number of women. Twenty per cent of the men and 4% of the women reported they would also lie if asked about a positive HIV test result [9].

Infidelity is not exclusive to men, but in many societies different preconceptions about male and female sexuality make women more likely than men to be faithful. In Thailand, for example, "a man's social status used to be measured according to the number of women he had," says Chantawipa Apisook who works with the women's organisation EMPOWER. "This attitude today is reflected in the acceptance of a man who openly keeps a 'minor wife' or who frequents bars, coffee shops or massage parlours [10]."

Research shows large numbers of men regularly or occasionally visit prostitutes for sex. A 1989 study in Birmingham in the United Kingdom estimated that between 8% and 22% of local men have visited prostitutes. Approximately one-third of the men were married and two-thirds had a regular sex partner other than a prostitute [11].

According to Dr Geoff Foster, founder and president of Zimbabwe's Family AIDS Counselling Trust, "the unfaithful husband" is a major issue in any AIDS education session with women [12]. Many women refuse to acknowledge their partner's behaviour, because they feel powerless to change the situation. Denial means they are unable to take the first steps towards responding to their own risk of infection.

It takes two to be faithful. How effective are strategies based on fidelity messages in societies which continue to sanction different standards of sexual conduct for men and women? *Ministry of Health, Labour, Housing, Broadcasting and Information, St Lucia / St Lucian Artist Association*

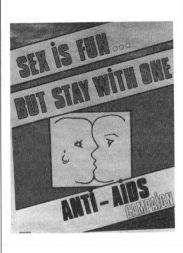

A Puerto Rican doctor found a similar difficulty. "When I start to talk about 'protection'...I am often confronted by silence. When I push the issue, and explain how condoms can protect, all the red flags go up. Some of these women know that their husbands are carrying on behind their backs...but they will

# Condom use - the catch 22

Norah, one of my friends, asked me for advice one day. She was worried that her husband might be infected with HIV, and pass it on to her. She knew that her husband often "met with" girlfriends at beer halls and hotels. She had never liked the fact but regarded it as inevitable. She had never mentioned to him that she knew about his girlfriends because this would make him angry.

I asked her whether she had thought of suggesting that they use condoms. Of course, she told me, but even the suggestion would cause problems. Her husband would either accuse her of infidelity, or charge her with accusing him of infidelity. He would become angry and not use the condom. If she asked him to use condoms when he went with girlfriends she would thereby reveal that she knew about them. This again would make him very angry. Had she talked with her husband, in general terms, about the problems of AIDS in the community, I asked. She said that she had tried to tell her husband how serious the disease was, but, like other men, he did not believe that AIDS existed in the area. We finally agreed that all she could really do was to try to talk to her husband once again about how common HIV infection is in the community, using a story about an imaginary friend who has been infected with HIV by her husband.

Norah loves her husband and does not want to leave him. Her children need their father and the family needs money for school fees, books and clothes. Her fears that he might contract HIV and might infect her are well founded. She is a well educated, mature woman in a responsible skilled job, but as the balance of power in her marriage lies with her husband, she is prevented from protecting herself from HIV.

**Wendy Holmes,** *Zimbabwe*

refuse to admit it. When I talk of 'protection' they are invariably confronted with the possibility of infidelity. That is the cultural Catch 22. Besides, they don't think it's lady-like to ask such things from their husbands....Believe me, we have a problem, but how do we convince women that they may be at risk when their denial systems kick into gear the moment you talk protection [13]."

Little research has been done on the distibution of HIV infection according to marital status or other partnership patterns. Polygamy, for example, is practised in parts of Africa and the Middle East. What is clear is that a traditionally polygamous family — where one man is married to several wives, and husband and wives have no other sexual partners — is no more at risk of HIV infection than a mutually and permanently monogamous couple. Some argue that polygamous marriages are less likely to lead to infidelity, making them a safer family unit from the point of view of HIV than a monogamous couple. However, if one person is unfaithful, the risks are magnified and affect the whole group. There may also be a risk when a new wife comes into the unit.

For women, the sexual partnerships which have generally been regarded as those involving least risk from HIV and AIDS are those with other women — with some justification, as there have been few reported cases of possible woman-to-woman transmission. But sexual

*Risks are attached to activities — sexual orientation is not in itself a protection*

orientation is not in itself a protection. Risks remain firmly attached to activities and thus oral sex, for example, is as risky for lesbian women as anyone else, as is injecting drug use [14].

## Changing patterns

The meaning and practice of marriage and other socially recognised forms of liaison are not cast in stone and are affected by wider social change. Many countries of the developing world are currently undergoing particularly traumatic social upheaval with urban communities expected to absorb close to 1 billion people between 1975 and the end of the century [15]. Eighty per cent of growth in population in the next few decades will be in cities, say the United Nations [16].

Worldwide, rapid urbanisation has always had a major impact on social organisation and patterns of sexual relationships. In some African cities, for example, rural polygamy has been transmuted into a pattern where married men may have "outside" or "informal" wives, with whom they have a relationship that is more stable than that of a girlfriend but which has no legal status. The Society for Women and AIDS in Africa (SWAA) distinguishes between formal polygamy where a man has "several legal wives" and informal polygamy where a man has "one legal wife but other women friends who depend on him" [17].

For many, the move to the city is a flight from increasing rural poverty. Often undertaken by one partner alone, even if only temporarily, it disrupts the stability of existing relationships. Men looking for work may be separated from their wives for months at a time. At the same time, "Many women who leave their villages to find work in the city, especially those without formal education, find themselves alienated without the extended family and village community support, and resort to prostitution for economic survival. This is a universal and age-old dilemma for poor, uneducated, urban women," says Edda Ivan-Smith, a development journalist [18]. "Women sex workers [in Thailand]...are generally young, aged between 15 and 20 and from rural communities," says Jon Ungphakorn, director of the Thai Volunteer Service. "Most...have knowingly entered the industry because of various pressures and a high sense of obligation towards their families. They may be the sole family members in a position to clear family debts, or to create a better life for their families, or to enable younger brothers and sisters to obtain an education beyond primary school....Others may have been through a broken marriage, and may have a child to provide for...", he

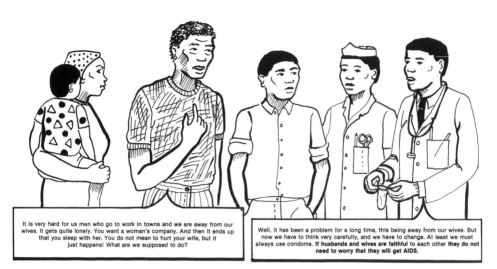

It is very hard for us men who go to work in towns and we are away from our wives. It gets quite lonely. You want a woman's company. And then it ends up that you sleep with her. You do not mean to hurt your wife, but it just happens! What are we supposed to do?

Well, it has been a problem for a long time, this being away from our wives. But now we have to think very carefully, and we have to change. At least we must always use condoms. **If husbands and wives are faithful to each other they do not need to worry that they will get AIDS.**

adds [19].

Some traditional sexual practices may also be significant in the spread or containment of the HIV epidemic. SWAA has called for an intensive health education campaign mobilising opinion leaders, local chiefs, religious authorities and politicians to alert people to the risks associated with some customary practices [20].

Education and counselling in some Zambian communities has meant changes in some practices. Traditionally, in many parts of Zambia, the family of a deceased spouse has the obligation to prepare the bereaved man or woman for re-marriage. This "cleansing" was usually done by a family member having sexual intercourse with the widow or widower. Today, while the social responsibility remains, non-sexual activities have been introduced to denote cleansing [21].

*AIDS education messages need to be firmly rooted in reality. This Zimbabwean book recognises that migration to the cities in search of work splits up families and affects people's relationships and sexual practices. "AIDS: Let us fight it together"/Women's Action Group, Harare, Zimbabwe*

## Motherhood

One major obstacle for women who wish to protect themselves against HIV infection is the desire to have a child. Safer sex — non-penetrative or condom-protected — presupposes sex without conception.

Decisions about motherhood are not taken in a vacuum. Every society, to a greater or lesser extent, accords status and respectability to women as childbearers. Childless women face stigma in many cultures; sometimes the penalty is desertion or divorce. But whatever the personal or social imperatives that govern motherhood, they will not vanish with the threat of AIDS. "The process by which decisions are made about using condoms (and other contraceptives) is related to a complex mixture of social, economic and cultural influences that

*Safer sex presupposes sex without conception*

*There is still a long way to go before the condom rescues the majority of women from the risk of STDs or AIDS, let alone pregnancy*

promote the role of motherhood for a woman, even when she knows she might already be infected with HIV," says US anthropologist Dr Dooley Worth [7].

In Kinshasa, Zaire, for example, condom use and sexual behaviour have been monitored since January 1988 in 175 couples where one partner is infected. Despite the risk of HIV infection, the desire to have children is the single most common reason for not using condoms. Among people who did not want a child, condom use was consistently very high [8]. Chapter 4 explores in more detail the issues involved in childbearing for HIV-positive women.

## The condom option

Lifelong fidelity or chastity may appear increasingly attractive options in the era of AIDS, but little evidence suggests that either is any more likely to be sustained. Where patterns of sexual behaviour have changed, having fewer partners or practising serial monogamy have been the more favoured options.

Some people are also turning to condom use as a result of AIDS education campaigns. Laboratory studies show that condoms prevent the passage of HIV. Used properly they provide the best available protection against HIV infection and studies show decreased levels of HIV infection among men and women who use them consistently. According to one of the world's major distributors, the International Planned Parenthood Federation (IPPF), condom use in some developing countries is rising dramatically.

In the North, condom use has also increased. For example, after public education campaigns in France, Switzerland and the United Kingdom, reported condom use and actual condom sales increased by between 5-20%, at least for a time [22]. Social marketing has helped — the 1990s "designer-condom" commercials feature young, good-looking couples — but there remains much to be done to improve the condom's image. Access, too, is improving in the North. Condoms are no longer sold under the counter in men's barber shops, but can be bought in supermarkets or from machines in women's toilets in bars, restaurants and student residences.

Increases in condom use, however, must be seen in the context of previous levels of use. "There is still a long way to go before the condom rescues the majority of women(or men)from the risk of STDs or AIDS, let alone pregnancy," says Marge Berer, a writer on women and AIDS. " Only 13% or less of women of childbearing age, married or in a union, surveyed in 56 developing countries in the 1970s and 80s, said they used condoms for contraception.In48 of those countries,

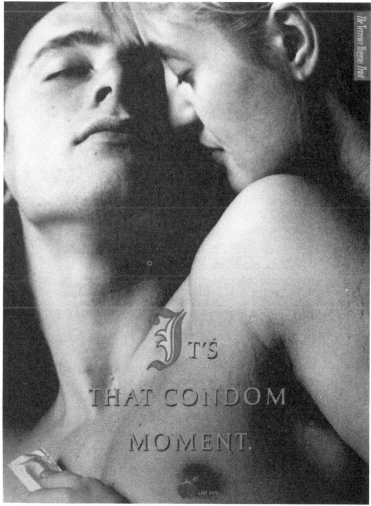

IT'S
THAT CONDOM
MOMENT.

Passion killers no longer. Safer sex campaigns are shifting away from attempts to scare people into protecting themselves, which many ignore, to approaches that emphasise the erotic. *The Terrence Higgins Trust, London, UK*

the figure was 5% or less. In all of the African and Middle Eastern countries surveyed, only 1% or less of the women used condoms for contraception [23]. While the figures are higher in some industrialised countries, they are almost all below 20% among women of childbearing age, with the notable exception of Japan," she adds [24].

In many parts of the world, people, particularly women, are still unaware of the existence of condoms or too poor to purchase them. One study of access to condoms in an area of rural Uganda, found that the majority of people had never used them, and about 15% had never heard of them [25]. In Senegal, women in the poorest communities surviving on prostitution find that the cost of a single condom on sale commercially is some two-thirds of the price they can charge for sex [26]. There is a great need for free or subsidised supplies and most

*In many parts of the world, women are still unaware of the existence of condoms, or too poor to purchase them*

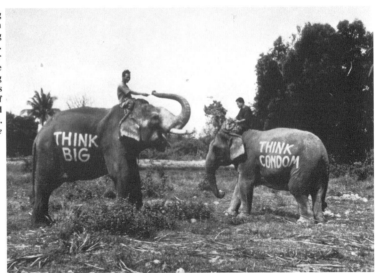

Condom campaigning on a grand scale in Thailand. But thinking big needs big resources. Supplies from donor agencies are inadequate and in 48 developing countries in the 1970s and 80s, less than 5% of married couples used condoms.
*Gemini News Service*

developing countries depend on Western donor agencies for this. The United States Agency for International Development (USAID) supplies half a billion condoms to the developing world every year — one-third of the total currently used. It is not even equivalent to one condom per year for each man aged 15 to 49 [27]. Dr Samuel Okware, former head of Uganda's AIDS Control Programme, commented that USAID's donation of two million condoms to Uganda in 1988 was "not enough for even a third of the adult population to swing into action once" [28].

"To promote condoms as a long-term contraceptive solution, family planning providers would need an unlimited supply," says Marge Berer. "Because many developing countries do not have such a supply and experience acute shortages, international family planning recommendations state that people at risk should continue to use their chosen method of contraception — using condoms for protection from STDs/HIV in addition when they are available," she adds [29].

For many women, the main reason for not using condoms as protection against HIV is the same reason they do not use them to protect against unwanted pregnancy: the need for their partner's agreement. "The woman is the party responsible for requesting their use in heterosexual relationships," says Brazilian anthropologist Jane Galvao. "The woman has to make rubbers erotically appealing (here they are known as the 'sheath of Venus', which has obvious feminine overtones); the woman has to choose the best time, place etc and 'beg' her partner to use condoms; and after she has done everything the purveyors of safe sex and wise health practices have encouraged, then he is the one who can say 'no' [30]."

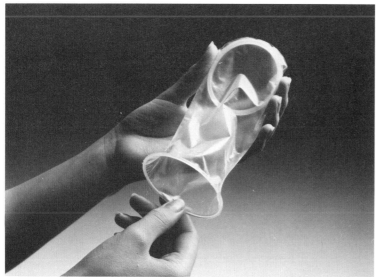

The female condom, due for approval in 1991.Will it bring more choice for women or more responsibility?

## The female condom

A new device being developed, the female condom, has the major advantage that its use can be controlled directly by women, freeing them, at least to some degree, from the need to negotiate safer sex. Family planners point out that a man will know when a woman is using a female condom, thus not entirely removing the problem of possibly uncooperative partners. The female condom is inserted like a contraceptive diaphragm or cap and held in place by an outer ring. Still under investigation in the United States and Europe, it is not yet available for use [31].

Initial trials suggest it could provide an important alternative to the male condom and that exposure to semen is significantly less than with the male condom because of fewer leaks or slippages. The female condom may also have a longer shelf-life and be stronger because it is made of polyurethane, not latex. Nor is it susceptible to deterioration with oil-based lubricants, one of the commonest reasons why traditional condoms break. If further study confirms these results, the female condom could prove to be at least as effective as the male condom at preventing HIV transmission. Companies developing the female condom estimate it will be available in the United States and Europe by the end of 1991 [32]. Pilot acceptability studies are also being carried out in some developing countries. Some AIDS educators are wary, however, that the new condom will place all the responsibility for protection upon women.

## Viricides

If using condoms is not possible, an alternative for women might be to use a diaphragm or cap together with a contraceptive spermicide such as Nonoxynol 9 (NO9) which is also a viricide — a virus-killer. Many health educators and some national AIDS programmes have recommended using NO9 or other viricides in addition to condoms for greater protection against HIV [33].

Although tests show NO9 kills HIV in the laboratory, it has not been possible to demonstrate the same effect when it is used by women. There is also concern that, because it is a detergent, NO9 can cause irritation in men and women which might therefore increase the risk of HIV transmission. A 1989 Canadian study found that more than half of a group using condoms lubricated with NO9 experienced side-effects such as irritation, numbness and burning [34]. One Kenyan study of 98 uninfected women found that NO9 was ineffective in preventing HIV transmission when used in vaginal suppositories and contraceptive sponges, and may have been associated with increased rates of genital ulcers and associated HIV infection, although it was also associated with a decrease in gonorrhoea [35]. However, both these studies were carried out with women working in the sex industry, who were at higher risk of other STDs and who used NO9 more frequently than the average user would. Research is now under way to develop alternative non-detergent viricides.

## NEGOTIATING SAFER SEX

Condoms are only part of safer sex. Suggesting alternatives to intercourse, such as oral sex or mutual masturbation, can also pose problems. "In my experience it's even more difficult talking about the non-penetrative option. Why? I think that at least part of the answer lies in the fact that, right from the first mention of sex at school, we make assumptions about what a sexual encounter between a man and a woman actually is," says Ceri Hutton, policy development officer at the UK National AIDS Trust [36]. "There is a well established 'male' sense of what it is to 'have sex', generally meaning penile-vaginal intercourse," agrees researcher Gloria Mock. Other types of sexual pleasure are often thought to be immature or not wholly satisfying [37].

The pros and cons of condom use are a reflection of many of the larger issues surrounding sexual decision-making which family planning campaigners have faced for many years. Research with women worldwide reveals that many find decision-making about the when and how of sex rests very much with their partners, who frequently object to condoms. The prevailing norm, says Dr Mindy

Fullilove, a US psychologist and director of Multicultural Inquiry and Research on AIDS, is that men initiate sex and women respond, and that this leaves women at a disadvantage in any sexual negotiations. Women's bargaining power for condom use may be minimal or non-existent: "The power women have is to negotiate, plead, beg, while the man has the power to turn down and deny," says Brazilian anthropologist, Jane Galvao [38].

The reasons men give for not using condoms vary from inconvenience to lessening of pleasure. "Using condoms is not really natural...it is not pretty, it is not practical, it is not poetic," was one British man's comment [39]. But prostitutes in several countries say they know how to put a condom on a client before he becomes aware of it and men who do use condoms say they soon get used to them.

Resistance to condoms is not exclusive to men, however. For many women the connotations of condoms are a powerful disincentive. Condoms are not just seen as contraceptives or protection against sexually transmitted diseases, but are associated with promiscuity and

# "Condoms or cross your fingers"

Targeting women in safer sex campaigns will be of limited effectiveness, say the London-based Women, Risk and AIDS Project (WRAP), unless campaigns take account of the gender-based power relations which limit women's choices in sexual relationships. Interviews with some 500 women aged 16-21, showed that most of their sexual activity was ultimately determined by men, say WRAP researchers. Many young women said they had sexual intercourse when they would have enjoyed or preferred non-penetrative sex, which they were aware is a means of avoiding HIV infection. The reason for the apparent contradiction is that many women define sex to a large extent according to what they believe gives men sexual pleasure, i.e. penetration, and they fail to assert their own preferences.

One young woman explained that she and her boyfriend didn't talk about sex and she felt unable to tell him what she liked sexually. Another, when asked whether she found her sexual relationship satisfying or pleasurable, said: "Well,...in the sexual relationships I've had...it's never been like it is in the books, I'm sure it could have been a lot better but, yeah, it was okay."

Men's control over sexual encounters extended beyond definitions of sex and sexual pleasure, say researchers. One young woman, when describing her first experience of condom use, explained that her boyfriend had been certain that the condom should be "blown up" first. In spite of the fact that she had strong doubts about this, she had allowed her views to be overridden on the assumption that "men knew better".

Some women rationalised their boyfriends' or their own opposition to condom use by convincing themselves that they were not at risk of either pregnancy or sexually transmitted diseases. Others feared losing their boyfriends or hurting their feelings and "employed a method based on 'condoms or cross your fingers' — using condoms when they were available or agreed upon, but going ahead anyway when they were not [61] ".

**Renée Danziger**, *United Kingdom*

*Ignorance about HIV is the most basic obstacle to protection for millions of women* furtive sex. "It is difficult for a woman to propose to her husband or male partner that safer sex be practised through condom use. As a wife she may be called a 'loose woman' or thought to be inferring the infidelity of her husband," say SWAA in their inaugural conference report [40]. According to Carmen Chavez of a Latino AIDS project in San Francisco, it is not easy to promote condoms among unmarried Latina women. Their use is equated with "whore-like" behaviour; the implication is that a woman carrying them is "available" for sex [41].

In a long-term relationship the sudden introduction of condoms where they have not been previously used can "threaten the trust that is implied (whether it exists or not)...[since] condoms for many individuals are symbols of extra-relationship activity. The subconscious message their use delivers is: 'You are not the only one with whom I am having sex'....It is the avoidance of such feelings that constitutes the major obstacle to condom use," says US anthropologist Dr Dooley Worth [42].

## THE POWER TO CHOOSE

Ignorance about HIV is the most basic obstacle to protection for millions of women worldwide. A 16-year-old woman working in the brothels of Pattaya in Thailand was asked what she would do if she suspected a client had HIV. She replied that she would make sure he had a good bath [43]. Primary health care workers have long known that low levels of literacy and income among women are associated with poor maternal and child health. It would be surprising if the same did not hold true for AIDS risk reduction.

### Information: access and action

Information about HIV is not available to many women living in areas with little health service provision. For many others the information may exist but circumstances deny them access. According to one Indian researcher, AIDS education will fail unless it acknowledges that many women are in a communications "purdah" or seclusion [44], beyond the reach of messages addressed to them.

Low levels of female literacy are a primary obstacle in many countries. "Empowerment cannot happen out of nothing. In our society most women are illiterate which makes spreading information about AIDS very much more difficult....The African woman is held back by economic dependence and significant socio-cultural burdens: religious, cultural and ethnic taboos which make discussion of some issues out of the question...", commented a delegate at the 1990 SWAA conference [45].

# Cultural constraints on choices: India

Epidemics are by definition hard to control. Coping with an epidemic based on sexual behaviour when it is a subject rarely discussed is even harder. And in India sex is the biggest secret of them all. It wasn't always so, as the explicit stone sculptures at Khajuraho testify. Even the Kamasutra — dubbed the most comprehensive treatise on sex ever compiled — is of Indian origin. Yet over the last few hundred years, different cultural influences and changing social conditions have combined to put sex into hiding.

Homosexuality officially does not exist. "Come with me one night and I'll show you at least three well-known men trying to make contact," challenges Ashok Row Kavi, a Bombay-based journalist and publisher of India's first magazine for homosexuals. Most homosexuals are married, often have children and lead double lives. In some cases the wife may know but she'll go along with it for the sake of preserving the marriage and thereby her identity in society.

Sexually transmitted diseases (STDs) are as prevalent in India as anywhere in the world, but among the thousands of voluntary agencies in the country today hardly any work in the area of STD prevention. Prostitution is big business, yet although 300,000 women take to prostitution every year, they have no union or representative body.

Both men and women suffer from the prevailing sexual morality, yet women bear the brunt of it. Virginity in an unmarried woman is automatically assumed while men are supposed to be "experienced" before marriage. The dichotomy confuses men as well. Visiting a prostitute is an option before marriage and in a relationship grown stale through lack of privacy, too many children and too little money, a prostitute remains an occasional luxury to be enjoyed — usually without condoms.

"Lack of condom use is probably one reason why a very high proportion of the [prostitute] population suffers from STDs," explains Dr Sundar, a psychiatrist who has worked with prostitutes in Madras. The women report that most men do not use condoms because they say it lessens sexual pleasure. The woman herself has no power to demand its use as she is often uneducated, poor and dominated by the police-politician-pimp nexus that controls the trade. "So they are constantly reinfected and obviously pass the infection on to the clients, but until the men are educated about STDs — especially HIV now — it is no use talking of intervention. Intervention must start with the male client," says a Madras-based social worker.

One reason for the casual attitude towards STDs could be the discovery of penicillin almost on the heels of STD entry into the country. "Europe had a much longer history of STDs before a cure was discovered so people learnt to take precautions. That culture completely by-passed us. That is why heterosexual transfer of HIV will be the biggest mode of transfer," Sundar concludes.

Condoms are also largely seen as a contraceptive for family planning and therefore find no place in a prostitute-client relationship. There are difficulties over their use even within a marriage. "The basic problem is disposal," admits Dr Balakrishna of the Family Planning Association of India. "Villagers don't have flushing systems, they don't even have toilets. Besides they all sleep in one room — parents, children, grandparents, perhaps an unmarried brother or sister. When sex itself is an act of stealth, the question of using a condom doesn't arise!"

Despite the wide differences in caste and class, education and affluence, women throughout India have in common a lack of access to factual information about sex, and limited options for behaviour. Sex education in schools is conspicuous by its absence.

Veena is an accounts executive with an advertising firm in Madras. "The first time my husband and I went all the way was the night we were married. Ours was a love marriage: he educated in the West; I, a post-graduate working woman. Both liberal, both progressive but when it came to sex...we just couldn't seem to find a way to enjoy it and yet not risk pregnancy. He didn't want to use a condom, I didn't want to go on the pill and my doctor ruled out the use of an IUD for somebody who hadn't >>

had a child yet. In fact she tried to persuade us to have a baby immediately, even though I was barely 22. 'Space the second', she advised. That's exactly how it worked out though I wish I had been more careful in the first place. I just didn't know how to discuss it or with whom."

Viji, daughter of an affluent landowner in rural Karnataka, also found she had no options. She left school at 17 to be married to a 22-year-old engineer in Bangalore. "I had my first child at 18, two others in the next three years and went through a sterilisation as well, all by the time I was 22. Contraceptives? What for? We were sure we didn't want any more children, so an operation was the best thing. Maybe we could have used something before our first child, maybe if he had said something about it. ...I just didn't know anything and I couldn't even have dreamt of talking about sex with him at that time."

In the few cases where couples agree to space children, the woman normally gets an IUD fitted. But this decision is often something the elders in the family have to support — and many do not. "Why space children at all? Have them when you are young and get operated once and for all," insists one village elder in Alampundi. The young pregnant girl sitting beside her giggles shyly but nods in agreement. And what of delaying the first? "People will think I am impotent if we don't have a child in a year," laughs her husband.

Women in village societies appear to be marginally better off in some ways. "At least they know what the sexual act involves, and close relationships — especially among peer groups — ensure a certain amount of discussion, even among women. But the discussions never occur between sexes, reinforcing the basic divide," argues social worker Venkatesh. "Options? You get married, have intercourse the first night, conceive within the next couple of months, have another three or four children in the next few years and perhaps get sterilised at the end of it all. What is there to discuss? It is understood that the man may sleep around. That's all right as long as he looks after his family. If he gets infected with an STD, he gets himself a shot of penicillin at the nearest private clinic to maintain anonymity and then it's back to normal."

**Shyamala Nataraj,** *India*

Domestic isolation is another significant factor. In rural areas in the developing world, women work long, hard days with little opportunity to benefit from public information and education programmes. In urban areas, women are more likely than men to remain in the home beyond the reach of public or workplace health campaigns. Isolation is most intense for those furthest from the dominant culture. In the United States for example, among immigrant Mexican American women, those who were least integrated into society had the lowest AIDS knowledge [46].

One place where counselling may often be offered to women about HIV risks is the pre-natal clinic — but those most in need are the least likely to benefit. "In New York in our communities", says Sallie Perryman, of the AIDS Institute of the New York State Department of Health, talking about black women in Brooklyn, "thirty per cent of the women never get pre-natal care. The time they come to the hospital is for delivery. What kind of counselling can you give by that time [47]?" Some women get no information on AIDS until after they have had their children. "Women are often infected without knowing it. Sometimes the first time they do know it is when their sick baby is diagnosed," says Professor Constance Wofsy, co-director of AIDS activities at San Francisco General Hospital [48].

Getting information about AIDS is a crucial first step, but changing behaviour is an even greater hurdle. Many women who are aware of the dangers of HIV-infection are constrained in their ability to use information to their advantage. Women who appear too knowledgeable or assertive about sexual matters may find their character called into question [49]. Yet a change to no and low-risk sex requires a woman to state what she wants and why, and to get her partner to cooperate. "The level of communication about sex and sexuality in any relationship, as well as actual practice, is often socially, rather than individually, defined," says writer Marge Berer [50]. US anthropologist Dr Dooley Worth sees "relative sexual equality " as essential for any AIDS prevention programme which relies upon women's sexual decision-making [51].

*The level of communication about sex in a relationship is often socially, rather than individually, defined*

## THE POVERTY FACTOR

Female poverty often brings with it an increased risk of HIV infection through restricted access not only to health information, but also to health services such as STD treatment and condom supplies. Apart from the fact that women on low incomes cannot afford condoms, often their negotiating position with sexual partners is undermined by economic dependence.

Poverty affects attitudes to risk-taking in other complex ways. Unless AIDS is seen in the context of wider issues, educators fear the AIDS message will fall on deaf ears. Marie St Cyr, a counsellor working in inner-city New York, asks: "If the only ways of escape people have are through drugs and sex — which offer a rare chance to feel like a complete human being — and both of these are very closely linked with AIDS, then what hope is there of addressing the issue of AIDS prevention without addressing the underlying issue of what people are trying to escape from [52]?" When too much energy is expended on basic survival issues, people tend to ignore a disease which might not materialise for years [53]. Too many contending issues of poverty can crowd AIDS out. "This AIDS is nothin'. I gotta worry where I'm gonna sleep tonight and whether he's gonna beat me," said one US woman who was pregnant and had HIV. She was on methadone maintenance (the treatment for people addicted to heroin), and lived in an abandoned building with a violent partner [54].

"A lack of economic, social, cultural, sexual and technological options combine to lead vulnerable women to concentrate on addressing the more immediate risks in their lives: poverty, homelessness and the frequent disruption of socioeconomic support systems," concludes one study looking at resistance to condom use among women at high risk [55].

## Prostitution: dangerous women or women in danger?

The dangers of economic dependence are most acute for women who have never had the chance to develop skills needed to earn a living, including many women who marry early and later face a breakdown in their marriage. In extreme economic hardship, many women may turn to prostitution to support themselves and their children. The term prostitution covers a wide range of circumstances but is sometimes wrongly applied. Boundaries are very often blurred: exchanging sex for money or material goods — clothing, gifts — may be part of many relationships which neither partner regards as prostitution.

Nevertheless, the global business of prostitution — the selling of sex to a (usually) male client — graphically illustrates the ways in which economic and social circumstances influence women's exposure to risk. Women in the sex industry live and work in very different conditions around the world and the degree of control they exert over their own lives varies dramatically with these circumstances. An educated New York call girl living in her own apartment and selling sex to clients on her own terms is in a stronger position to refuse practices she knows may endanger her health. Many of the world's poorest women are not. In some countries, the extremely high HIV prevalence among groups of women working as prostitutes reveals just how closely AIDS tracks poverty. "At the end of 1989 around 10% of low-income sex workers were infected...infection among higher-income sex workers averaged at around 2%," reports Jon Ungphakorn, director of the Thai Volunteer Service [56].

*Around 10% of low-income sex workers were infected compared with 2% of higher-income sex workers*

Prostitution is an integral part of the formal and informal economies of countries worldwide. It can be big business — although not usually for the workers — and tends to be symptomatic of economic inequality rather than uniform poverty in a society [57]. In Thailand the sex industry has flourished during the past three decades of successful national development and economic growth and is estimated to serve tens of thousands of Thai men and foreign tourists. Some European, Japanese and US travel agents offer package holidays which cater specifically for sexual gratification. Thai women demonstrating in Bangkok in 1987 claimed that the Thai government spent 20 times more each year on tourism promotion than it did on its AIDS prevention activities [58].

*For many women it is a choice between survival that day or risking HIV infection*

Many of the women most at risk, particularly in the poorest countries of the developing world, live in extreme poverty and are unlikely to have information about safer sex. Condoms are very often unavailable or unaffordable. Clients may be unwilling to use them and prepared to go elsewhere or to pay more for unprotected sex.

Telling a woman she must refuse to put herself at risk through unprotected sexual intercourse — when the alternative may be that she is unable to feed herself or her child that day — seems to be asking the impossible. "For many women it is a matter of either possible HIV infection or survival for that particular day...inevitably they choose survival at the risk of infection," says Dr John Chikwem discussing a risk-reduction programme with Nigerian women working as prostitutes [59].

In richer, industrialised countries women in the sex industry tend to have greater access to information and condoms. Regular condom use results in low incidence of STDs, including HIV, for sex workers who have no other risk factors. In addition, oral sex and manual stimulation, low-risk and effectively no-risk activities respectively, are the most commonly demanded sexual services from street prostitutes in the United States [60].

## Individual choice?

Individuals' sexual relationships may be the most personal and intimate part of their lives, yet they are built on and reflect society's most fundamental norms. Social and economic circumstances, plus deep-rooted and widespread beliefs about the passive nature of female sexuality and the values ascribed to motherhood, combine in many societies to undermine women's control over their own bodies and — literally, in the case of AIDS — their own destinies.

# CHAPTER 4

# HIV INFECTION, REPRODUCTION AND MOTHERHOOD

"Often I find myself in the role of informal HIV-counsellor, expected to answer questions about risk behaviour, about life and its meaning, about death. These are big demands to put on anyone. ...Many times I have had the dubious pleasure of being treated as a health educator, while lying on some hospital couch, longing to be small, to be 'weak', to be cared for as a patient...", says Amanda Heggs, a British woman in her early thirties, diagnosed with HIV in 1986 in Denmark. She continues, "I believe...many...problems arise because, among other things, it is all too easy for female nurses (many of whom are in my own age-group) to identify themselves with me. Faced with a female, middle-class, non-injecting drug user who is HIV-positive, it is no longer possible to deny their potential vulnerability to HIV. An auxiliary nurse told me that, the last time I was hospitalised, she had been unable to come into my room, because she was waiting for the result of her own antibody test, and just could not bear to be confronted with a woman who was HIV-positive [1]".

## HIV DISEASE IN WOMEN

In industrialised countries, because relatively few women developed AIDS in the early days of the epidemic, systems, services and public consciousness of the issue all grew up around AIDS as a disease for men — generally gay men. Today, the proportion of women affected worldwide is growing fast, but awareness about the ways in which HIV affects women and the services they need lags behind.

In the mid-1980s, much information about the course of HIV infection and the spectrum of related disorders in women was based on assumptions derived from long-term studies of AIDS in men. Since then, it has become evident that HIV disease in women differs in some ways. According to Dr Constance Wofsy, co-director of AIDS activities at San Francisco General Hospital, "We desperately need information about the mortality, morbidity and special effects of HIV/AIDS on women...there are obviously sex-related issues that need specific attention, links with cervical cancers etc — and we must begin to seriously investigate these [2]."

The basic course of HIV infection and disease is the same for men and women. Doctors increasingly characterise it in four stages (see

Chapter 1): a mild bout of illness often follows infection; that is *Early US* followed by a period without symptoms of, on average, 10 years, *statistics* although laboratory tests show that the immune system is weakening *suggested that* during this time; symptoms such as skin problems and oral thrush then *HIV-positive* appear; these are followed by more serious symptoms such as night *women were* sweats, weight loss and diarrhoea or major illnesses such as the severe *diagnosed* form of pneumonia, *pneumocystis carinii* (PCP) or an aggressive *later and died* tumour *Kaposi's sarcoma* (KS), which can involve several organs but *more quickly* primarily the skin. At this stage of illness AIDS is diagnosed. *than men*

Early manifestations of HIV infection in women may also include persistent gynaecological complaints such as cervical inflammation, vaginal thrush and possibly pelvic inflamatory disease (PID). Genital warts are also more commonly detected among HIV-positive women and are linked to an increase in cervical disorders including cancer [3]. Frequency of cervical abnormalities increases as women begin to show symptoms of HIV infection [4]. As a result, wherever possible, HIV-positive women are advised to have regular cervical smears. Some doctors suspect that these gynaecological disorders are also more aggressive and recurrent in HIV-positive women and require different and more extensive treatment than in HIV-negative women [5]. Pregnancy may complicate early diagnosis in women. Symptoms such as persistent vaginal thrush, shortness of breath and fatigue, which can result from HIV infection, are also side-effects of pregnancy in some HIV-negative women [6].

Among people with AIDS, PCP is detected more frequently in industrialised countries while African studies have found that a major manifestation of AIDS is diarrhoea and wasting. In one Nairobi study, it occurred in more than 80% of women who died [7]. US studies have shown that HIV-positive women are relatively unlikely to develop KS, which typically affects homosexual men with AIDS. Scientists now think that KS might be sexually transmitted [8]. In Uganda, recent research suggests HIV-associated KS, which differs from the milder KS endemic in Africa (which is not believed to be sexually transmitted), is increasing among men and women [9].

## "Women die faster, it's a disaster"

"Women die faster, it's a disaster", claimed US women activists at the Sixth International Conference on AIDS in 1990. Early statistics from the United States suggested that HIV-positive women were diagnosed later and died more quickly after diagnosis than men. This is partly because, as indicated earlier in this dossier, many women lack access to information and health care, and is partly a reflection of the common belief in the industrialised world that only certain "risk groups", such as prostitutes or drug users, are vulnerable. "Carmen...lost precious time", says US AIDS worker Kathe Karlson, "because doctors didn't diagnose her early on. Chronic vaginal infections and a sore throat started over eight years ago. Although doctors never mentioned HIV to her, she decided to take the test in 1987. She was positive [10]." Researchers feel strongly that doctors and others need guidelines to ensure timely recognition and management of gynaecological diseases both in HIV-positive women and in those at risk [11].

One study in New York State found that women, the majority of whom were black and Latina drug users or partners of drug-using men, were already very ill when they came forward for medical help. On average, women suffered nearly 60 weeks of ill health before seeking medical care, compared with just 24 weeks for men [12]. Black women and injecting drug users had the shortest survival times of all [13].

Although symptoms in men and women may be somewhat different, with proper and timely diagnosis and access to medical care, the medical picture of AIDS in women is not inherently better or worse than that for men. "A lot of women in the United States find out their HIV status when they're being diagnosed with an illness [caused by the virus]," says Katie Bias, herself HIV-positive. "I believe that at least part of the reason why women don't live as long as men after HIV diagnosis is because they've had no early intervention — no advice on immune system modulation, changing diet, stopping drinking or getting enough sleep and exercise — they don't do any of this because they don't think they're at risk....A gay white male goes into a doctor's office with certain symptoms and he gets an HIV test; a woman walks in with the same symptoms and they don't even consider it...[14]."

In those parts of the world, largely developing countries, where the commonest means of transmission is through heterosexual sex, health professionals may be less likely to misdiagnose HIV-related symptoms in either men or women. Nevertheless, in these countries, women's access to health care is often limited. Women's responsibilities and limited access to money or transport can mean less opportunity to travel to a health clinic — opportunities which may be further reduced by the obligations of working or taking care of other family members who are sick (see Chapter 6).

The gender gap in health care is not merely a phenomenon of AIDS. For example, according to the World Health Organization (WHO) "even if exposure to malaria is equal between men and women, women do not have the same chance of receiving adequate care during a malaria episode. First, unlike men, women are mostly engaged in more than one activity. Second, within the household, they are traditionally called on to tend to the needs of other sick family members. Third, when women become ill, there are usually few other household members willing or able to care for them. The result is that women tend to allow themselves less time off during disease episodes and are less likely to seek or obtain adequate care [15]".

# Women's access to clinical trials: the United States

Many drugs for HIV remain experimental but unless people are included in clinical trials, they have no access to such potentially life-saving treatment. In the United States, the majority of women with HIV/AIDS are black or Latina. For many, either they or their partners have a history of injecting drug use. Black and Latino people, and women, injecting drug users and children are all under-represented in experimental drug trials. According to the US AIDS treatment registry, 35% of people with AIDS in New York City are black but only 10% of those enrolled in government-sponsored trials are [65]. Drug users have been traditionally excluded from clinical trials because they are seen as unreliable.

In an attempt to widen access, US public health officials have now endorsed "Parallel Track" programmes for those who otherwise would be unable to take part in standard clinical trials. These locally run programmes are both easier for many to get to and less likely to inspire fear and suspicion. For women particularly, they may overcome problems of lack of transport and child-care provision.

Access to drug trials for women has also been restricted for another reason — because of the potential risk of birth defects should they become pregnant. More than half the US government drug trials still exclude women of childbearing age, and most of the others encourage women to be sterilised before participating, according to ACT UP New York, the activist group lobbying for more and broader clinical research. Activists argue that women should be allowed to take part in trials if they sign an agreement to use barrier contraceptives and agree not to hold drug companies liable for any harmful effects to themselves or their children should they become pregnant [66].

The exclusion of women from most research programmes has been further challenged by the possibility that anti-viral drug treatment for mothers may also be the best way of protecting their babies from infection [67]. Trials to determine the safety of anti-viral drugs such as zidovudine (commonly known as AZT) for pregnant women and their foetuses are now under way [68]. Anecdotal reports of women taking controlled doses of zidovudine during pregnancy have suggested no harmful effects on foetal development [69].

Participation in trials depends on more than being medically eligible. In practice, co-operation means long interviews, frequent blood tests and visits to universities or hospitals. "The point is that trials require someone to come very frequently; to keep to a tight schedule; and to be unencumbered by [children]. That's extremely inconvenient and just as special efforts have to be made to reach injecting drug users — such as pay incentives or whatever — the only way to include women in trials is to go out after them. I don't think there is any more to it than that," says Professor Constance Wofsy of San Francisco General Hospital [70].

Some people doubt that much can be done to redress the balance between those with and those without access to trials and health services generally, without other more fundamental changes taking place. "If you have a legacy of never being concerned with a community in terms of their health >>

care [and] if you haven't made the investment in that area — and then you have an epidemic like AIDS which demands labour- and resource-intensive efforts to maintain quality of life — you simply don't have the foundation for access to services. That is the major problem. ...Without efforts to bridge gaps for persons of colour, poor persons and particularly women of colour, the likelihood of 'parallel track' becoming a reality is dismal," comments Marie St Cyr, executive director of the Women's Action Resource Network in New York [71].

As far as developing countries are concerned, the gulf in provision is incomparably greater. "Clinical trials are desperately needed in the Third World, not only for the popular brands like zidovudine but also for the many and various herbs which are readily available," says Dr Elli Katabira of The Ugandan AIDS Service Organisation (TASO). "To accomplish this, genuine collaboration with the developed countries is required [72]." But collaboration must begin at the beginning, argues Dr Eustace Muhondwa of the University of Dar es Salam in Tanzania, with the deciding of priorities: too often North/South collaboration means the North defines the problem and then comes South "on safari" to collect data [73].

## DOES PREGNANCY AFFECT AN HIV-POSITIVE WOMAN?

During pregnancy a woman's immune system is weakened, making her more vulnerable to serious complications from several infections caused by bacteria, for example Salmonella, which causes a type of food poisoning; and viruses such as herpes simplex, the source of cold sores or genital herpes, and herpes zoster, which causes chicken pox or shingles. Because HIV infection attacks the body's immune system, scientists were initially concerned that pregnancy would automatically accelerate an infected woman's progression to AIDS. The current view, however, is that pregnancy does not affect the progression of HIV disease in those women who are infected but whose immune systems have not yet been compromised by HIV and who are still healthy [16]. Once the disease has progressed beyond this stage, however, the risks to the woman could be greater [17].

If a woman does develop infections characteristic of HIV infection during pregnancy, experts recommend that treatment be determined on a case-by-case basis. Not all drugs which might be used in therapy are safe for the foetus.

If a woman who injects drugs is pregnant, stopping drug-taking may slow progression of HIV-disease. There is thus a strong argument for expanded drug treatment programmes in countries where drug use is common, for both pregnant and non-pregnant women [18]. "Unfortunately, [in the US] drug treatment programmes dealing with the particular needs of women are rare, and few of the existing programmes are residential. There are only three methadone (a less harmful substitute for street heroin) treatment programmes in the United States that are specifically designed for pregnant women," says

US AIDS researcher Laurie Hauer [19]. A survey of 78 New York treatment programmes in 1989 found that 54% excluded pregnant women [12].

## MOTHER-TO-CHILD TRANSMISSION

A baby whose mother is HIV-positive can be infected in three ways: in the womb before birth (HIV has been detected in very early foetuses and in umbilical cord blood); possibly during delivery by the mother's infected blood or vaginal secretions; or, in a very few documented cases, from breastfeeding [21].

Most studies show that between 25% and 50% of all mothers with HIV-1 pass on the virus to their babies. Information on mother-to-child transmission of HIV-2 is scanty. Some experts say it may be "rare or absent" [22]. Others believe there is little evidence to suggest HIV-2 is necessarily different from HIV-1 [23].

In spite of some apparently contradictory findings, the similarities between transmission rates of HIV-1 from studies around the world are more striking than the differences, according to Professor

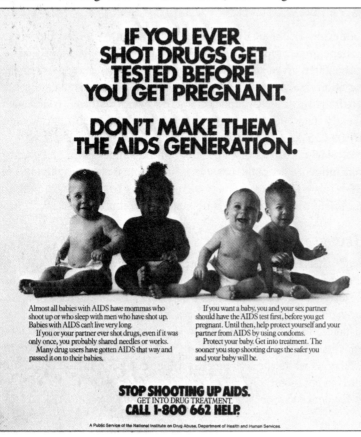

**IF YOU EVER SHOT DRUGS GET TESTED BEFORE YOU GET PREGNANT.**

**DON'T MAKE THEM THE AIDS GENERATION.**

Almost all babies with AIDS have mommas who shoot up or who sleep with men who have shot up. Babies with AIDS can't live very long.
If you or your partner ever shot drugs, even if it was only once, you probably shared needles or works.
Many drug users have gotten AIDS that way and passed it on to their babies.

If you want a baby, you and your sex partner should have the AIDS test first, before you get pregnant. Until then, help protect yourself and your partner from AIDS by using condoms.
Protect your baby. Get into treatment. The sooner you stop shooting drugs the safer you and your baby will be.

**STOP SHOOTING UP AIDS.**
GET INTO DRUG TREATMENT.
**CALL 1-800 662 HELP.**

A Public Service of the National Institute on Drug Abuse, Department of Health and Human Services

In the United States and Europe, sharing needles to inject drugs is a major route for HIV transmission. Women may be at risk from injecting or from sex with a drug-injecting partner — in either case their baby may be at the end of the line of infection: born with HIV. *National Institute on Drug Abuse, Department of Health and Social Services, US*

Breastmilk is nutritious and passes on a mother's protective antibodies against common infections to her infant. HIV has been transmitted in breastmilk only in the most unusual of circumstances and the World Health Organization advises mothers to protect their infants' health by breastfeeding.
*Nancy Durrell McKenna*

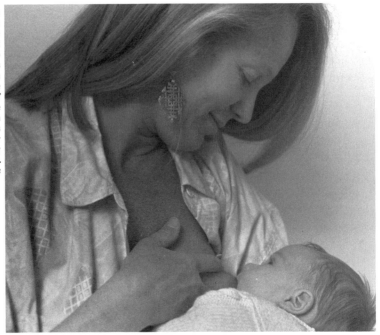

Catherine Peckham, a research co-ordinator of the European Collaborative Study of Perinatal (mother-to-child) Transmission — particularly given the different methods used in research and the variations in the health and circumstances of women studied. French [24], Italian [25] and Rwandan [26] studies, which all focused on women in early stages of infection, report mother-to-child transmission rates of 30%, 25% and 34% respectively.

Scientists suspect that the health of the mother during pregnancy may influence her child's chance of infection. If she has symptoms of HIV- related disease, she may be more likely to transmit the virus to her infant. However, there is no evidence to confirm this [27].

## Breast is still best

Fears that HIV might be transmitted by breastmilk have led to controversial guidelines on the subject from public health agencies. Researchers now believe that the handful of documented cases where mothers did transmit HIV by breastfeeding were atypical. In each instance, the mother had received infected blood during a blood transfusion immediately following birth and was therefore unusually infectious while she was breastfeeding because of high levels of the virus in her blood.

Evidence that breastmilk does not normally present a risk of HIV transmission comes from studies of HIV-positive mothers and their babies in Kinshasa, Zaire [28] and Haiti [29] and elsewhere. Breast and bottlefed babies of HIV-positive mothers did not differ in their likelihood of being HIV-positive.

Many doctors in the West still advise HIV-positive mothers to bottlefeed. The practice is, however, highly dangerous in developing countries, where bottlefed babies are on average twice as likely to die as breastfed babies from diseases caused by dirty water, unsterile bottles, and under-nourishment. In addition, formula feeds, unlike mother's milk, do not give babies immunity to certain diseases. WHO strongly urges that "particularly where the safe and effective use of alternatives is not possible, breastfeeding by the biological mother should continue to be the feeding method of choice, irrespective of HIV-infection status [30]".

## TO TEST OR NOT TO TEST ?

In some countries, the concern with possible mother-to-child transmission of HIV has led to pregnant women being offered the opportunity to test for the virus at ante-natal clinics. If the test proves positive, they are then able to make an early, informed decision as to whether to continue or terminate a pregnancy. If consent to such testing is to be truly voluntary and informed, it must be preceded by sensitive and appropriate counselling. It must also be accompanied by the assurance that a woman's health care will continue unaffected if she chooses not to take the test, or if the result is positive.

Even in such circumstances, testing has proved controversial. Those in favour argue that it benefits all women, whatever the result. Counselling, followed by a negative result, would allay any fears a woman might have about her HIV-status. If her result is positive, there is the opportunity for further counselling and better-informed medical care for any infections that might arise during pregnancy.

Interviews with women at one of the largest mother and child clinics in Brazzaville, Congo, found that the majority "show a very ambivalent attitude towards HIV-screening and recommendations which may be made depending on the results of the test", according to Dr M'pélé of the National AIDS Control Programme. Although many women interviewed felt a HIV-positive pregnant women should have an abortion, most said their individual choice would be to continue with pregnancy [31].

There are also concerns about the effectiveness of ante-natal testing in reaching women who would benefit most from it. Evidence from industrialised countries suggests that the women most at risk of HIV

*Loss comes in many forms — losing the ability to have a child can be as severe as losing a family member*

infection are least likely to recognise such a possibility or to take the test. Clinics which offer HIV testing only to women who acknowledge risk factors will overlook many who do not wish to reveal past risky behaviour. In a New York City study which offered testing to all women, only 40% accepted. All of those found positive described risk factors after receiving their test results which they had witheld in pre-test counselling [32]. In another US study, 1,000 women whose blood was anonymously tested for HIV were asked if they would like their test result. Only half of the 50 who admitted risk activity wanted to know their results, and they accounted for only 14% of those who were infected [33]. Similar findings have been reported in studies of men and women attending sexually transmitted disease (STD) clinics [34]. Reluctance to take the test has been linked to people's fear of knowing that they are HIV-positive or their anxiety about possible discrimination against them should their result become known.

Ultimately, health-care providers stress that women need HIV information and related prevention efforts before they become pregnant and before they are infected. Only then can the spread of HIV from mothers to infants be reduced [35].

## CHILDBEARING CHOICE

"For me one of the most difficult things to deal with has been the fact that we don't have any children," says Katie Bias, a US woman who is HIV-positive. Her husband, who has haemophilia, is also positive. "I was in a symposium on loss and grief and I thought I hadn't really 'lost' anyone. But it turns out that loss comes in many forms — and the loss of the ability to have a child is right up there with losing a family member. It's your potential....I'm experiencing the loss of someone who never existed but it's someone who I had always planned to get to know one day [36]."

When a woman finds she is HIV-positive while pregnant, whether this knowledge comes as a result of ante-natal testing or because she or her partner become ill, the stress she experiences is enormous. She has to deal at once with her own diagnosis as well as the possibility that her child might be infected. Pregnancy may be a time when she feels particularly vulnerable. "I live in the rural areas most of the time and sometimes visit my husband in town....He works in a factory in Harare....My husband told me he had this illness when I was pregnant with the last born," says one Zimbabwean woman. "[The doctor] explained this disease to me and I became frightened — especially when I realised that it could harm the baby I was carrying. My test was also positive. I have to accept all this — what else can I do [37]?"

Where abortion is a legal and safe option, a woman faces the often *Scientists* agonising decision over whether to continue or terminate her *cannot* pregnancy [38]. Not all of those who would wish to abort — because *pinpoint which* of the risk to the baby, the possible risks to themselves, and their *women are* potentially limited life -span — are able to. In many parts of the world *most likely to* abortion is not a legal — and therefore safe — option. For those who *transmit HIV* can and do decide to abort, an already painful choice may be made *to their foetus* more difficult by the fears that HIV arouses even in medical workers. One study in New York City found that 64% of clinics surveyed would not perform an abortion for an HIV-positive woman, violating city public health and anti-discrimination laws [39].

Many HIV-infected pregnant women who are counselled early enough to consider abortion decide to continue their pregnancy [40]. One second-time pregnant woman in the United States was admonished by a doctor for being irresponsible — at the time it was thought she had a 50% chance of infecting her baby. She replied that since her HIV diagnosis, those were "the best odds" she had heard [41].

According to Dr Janet Mitchell, an obstetrician at New York's Harlem Hospital, the medical profession's surprise about such reactions stems from an inability to see the situation from the women's perspective. "For many women, childbearing is seen as life-affirming in the face of poverty, drug use, racism, and perhaps the loss of other children to foster care or AIDS. In addition, even a 50% perinatal transmission rate is perceived by some women as an acceptable risk," says Laurie Hauer, a US AIDS researcher [42].

Children, or the prospect of having them, represent an investment in the future for many women and are a strong motivating force in their lives. "That is why many of these [HIV-positive] women choose to continue their pregnancies," says Dr Mitchell [43]. A study in Ireland among women infected with HIV through injecting drug use found a marked difference in attitude between those women who already had children and those with none. Women with children were much more likely to have thought ahead than those without children and had already made plans for what might happen if they became ill [44]. The same considerations influence women's decisions about whether to try to conceive if they are HIV-positive. A study in Kinshasa, Zaire found that many HIV-positive women were unwilling to sustain birth-control use, saying they desired a child [45].

North and South, women contemplating pregnancy can only consider the statistical risk that their child might become infected. The medical knowledge that might provide an assessment of individual risk is still not available — scientists cannot pinpoint which women are most likely to transmit HIV to their foetus or which babies are most susceptible [46].

Drugs that might prevent transmission of HIV are not yet available. Anti-viral drugs such as zidovudine (commonly known as AZT) are being tested but there is, as yet, no evidence that they prevent mother-to-child transmission [47]. Even if such drugs do become available, they will not be affordable for the majority of HIV-positive women.

Personal choice and medical risk are not the only factors influencing the decision whether to continue a pregnancy or plan one. Individual decisions reflect wide-ranging social and cultural expectations about motherhood and childbearing. US doctors report that many pregnant HIV-positive women who choose to have their child give as reasons their religious beliefs and family pressure. "In Latin America and the Caribbean a woman's role has generally been defined as a bearer of children," says Dr Ann Marie Kimball of the Pan American Health Organization [48]. This constrains her choices about continuing or terminating a pregnancy. In Chikankata, Zambia, about one in every three HIV-positive women tell the counsellor that it will not be possible for them to refuse to become pregnant again [49]. According to US doctor Janet Mitchell, when "society defines the primary function of a woman as bearing children, not bearing children makes that woman an abnormal part of that society. To change that focus on childbearing entails a re-education of every single member of that society [50]".

Where a woman and her partner agree together that they want a child, even though one or both of them has the virus, advice about how to minimise risks is invaluable. This includes learning to recognise when in the menstrual cycle she is most likely to get pregnant and using barrier contraception or avoiding intercourse at other times [51].

For women in the North who are HIV-negative but whose partners are positive, there may eventually be another hope. Some data now suggests that only the seminal fluid of infected men contains HIV, not the sperm cells. The search is on for viable ways to separate sperm from seminal fluid, to allow for safe, but expensive, artificial insemination (AI). In the meantime, some women are using donated sperm from artificial insemination agencies which screen for HIV.

Some AIDS educators have raised the possibility of developing a selective viricidal agent which would not kill human sperm and hence allow conception, but which would prevent infection by killing HIV. Most scientists consider the possibility of developing such a compound extremely unlikely [52].

Just as access to information is fundamental to HIV prevention for women, so a woman's decision over whether to continue with or plan a pregnancy in the light of an HIV diagnosis needs to be made in the context of all available information. The personal and ethical dilemmas regarding pregnancy and childbearing for HIV-infected women "are among the most difficult faced by any persons with HIV infection", says Peter Selwyn, a US doctor [53]. According to US AIDS researcher Laurie Hauer, "It is critical that health workers remain non-directive and non-judgemental when discussing pregnancy options [54]".

*Decisions regarding childbearing are among the most difficult faced by anybody with HIV infection*

## LIVING WITH HIV

AIDS is a social as well as a medical issue, and anyone with AIDS needs much more than purely medical support. Prejudice and blame all too often follow a diagnosis of HIV infection and may have severe social and economic ramifications. Drug therapy and medication may assist in alleviating the physical manifestations of HIV infection, but understanding and compassion, love and support are what help men and women with AIDS to see their future in terms of living with HIV rather than dying from it.

An AIDS diagnosis is associated by many people with "promiscuity". In a world which still sanctions different standards for men and women in many areas of life, this is a stigma which affects women particularly. In Romania, HIV-positive women with multiple partners were reportedly listed in official statistics as "prostitute" [55]. Ugandan medical social worker, Mary Amanyire Byangire, says "when a woman is sick with AIDS, she is automatically considered a 'loose' woman...regardless of [how] she got the infection [56]". One study in Zaire showed that although HIV-positive wives suspected that their husbands had transmitted the virus to them, the wives were held responsible for their illnesses and sent back to their families while the husbands began living with other women [57]. Women have often received more attention for their potential role as "infectors" of babies and men, than for the problems they face as people who have been infected, according to Dr Joanne Mantell of the AIDS research unit, New York City Department of Health, who adds "Headlines such as 'Nursing mother gives baby AIDS' and 'Infected [prostitute] spreads AIDS' contribute to the public perception of women as infectors [58]".

Women with HIV may lose social standing within their community. "We live in a male-dominated society," observes Noerine Kaleeba of The AIDS Service Organisation (TASO) in Uganda. "Often relatives will encourage a man who appears fit and well to leave his wife with AIDS and find another one, with no understanding

*A single
woman who is
diagnosed
HIV-positive
will find
herself in a
kind of social
death*

that he may pass the infection on to another woman. We have some clients who have lost a number of wives — and yet their relatives are still persuading the man to find a new one. People start to ask them: 'Why are you still alone?' [59]". Many women suffer economic consequences when an HIV-infected partner dies, and are shunned by relatives and others who might traditionally have provided for them and their children.

"A single woman who is diagnosed HIV-positive will find herself in the middle of a kind of 'social death'," says a young African woman with HIV. "In the first place she is a failure, unable to conform to the traditional laws of marriage. Secondly, life becomes much more difficult as the woman becomes very reluctant to make new friends...she fears she may pass on the virus through any sexual contact because many men refuse to use condoms. ...If she reveals her HIV status to her partner, this often leads to rejection...most people believe that people who contract HIV have been involved in bad, unacceptable sexual activities and HIV and AIDS are a shame and a disgrace...she fears that her children may be victimised as the offspring of a sinner and may suffer this social stigma for the rest of their lives [60]."

British woman Amanda Heggs contracted HIV from her partner, from whom she later separated. Since her diagnosis she feels she is seen as no longer "viable" by potential partners. "I have become very much the mother figure to whom my male friends bring their problems. Deep friendships evolve, which is gratifying, but I have a feeling that my sexual life is finished. At one point I did have a 'post-HIV' relationship with a man. I had imagined that carrying out safe sex in practice — no easy task, with the limited information available for HIV-positive women at that time — would be our greatest problem. I was wrong. I gradually discovered that my partner felt that I ought to be grateful to him, because he was 'courageous' enough to have a relationship with an HIV-positive woman. The worse thing was, I did start to feel grateful and to tolerate several things on his part which I would not otherwise have done, had I not been HIV-positive. HIV became a power factor [61]."

Sheila Gilchrist, an HIV-positive woman who founded the UK support group Positively Women, initially found no support when she was diagnosed. "When I left hospital I spent the next two years aimlessly drifting between male-oriented AIDS support groups and drug rehabilitation centres, neither of which remotely fulfilled my needs as an HIV-positive woman. I decided I had to find other women with whom I could relate and share all the emotions inside me.

"I put up posters with a phone number. Thankfully the phone calls came in and we started a support group. The relief and peace I experienced in sharing with other HIV-positive women gave me the the incentive to build Positively Women into an organisation. We now offer a range of counselling and support services for women who are infected or have AIDS or other associated conditions. We are still horrifed at the isolation and terror women are experiencing. One women telephoned us from a provincial city to say she hadn't been out of her house for six months, she was so afraid [62]."

*The worst thing about the virus is the feeling of isolation*

"The most horrible aspect of all this, for me, was not talking to anyone about it," says an HIV-positive woman who shared her story at the Women and AIDS Support Network Conference in Harare, Zimbabwe in 1989, and whose partner is also positive. "My partner did not want to face up to things in the way that that I did. It was just impossible to [explain how I was] feeling. It was too fresh, too raw a feeling. Not really a feeling at all, but many rolled together. [I went] from desperation to determination that I would cope and fight every bit of the way to make my life, our life together, good for as long as it lasted.

"This was some time ago. Now we have each developed our own way of handling the situation. I still need to talk to other people about my feelings in a way that he does not. ..I think the worst thing about the virus is the feeling of isolation and the fear that accompanies any step toward breaking the isolation....I am still afraid of people finding out I am HIV-positive, afraid of their reactions and prejudices, but I am no longer afraid of myself, nor of my relationship with the man with whom I share my life. We have our ups and downs, depressions and moments of panic, but we are living full and rewarding lives both as individuals and as a couple. I want to ask you all to help end the ignorance and panic that go with the words 'HIV-positive'. For many of us they are a fact of our lives [63]."

"There is hope," says a British woman who was infected through sex with her husband after 25 years of marriage. "The hope does not lie in miracle drugs, though they would undoubtedly be welcome and save lives, but in what those with HIV can do for themselves. As long as newspapers talk of AIDS and dying, people will feel they have nothing to lose by living in ignorance of their condition [64]."

# CHAPTER 5

# HIV DISEASE
# IN INFANTS

## SOURCES OF INFECTION

Mother-to-child transmission of HIV is by far the greatest source of infection for children. In most industrialised countries blood-to-blood infection, through the use of HIV-infected blood or blood products, has been very rare, although there have been significant outbreaks of infection in hospitals and institutions in Romania and the USSR.

Infected blood is a far less likely source of infection now than it was five years ago. For example, many children with haemophilia were infected in the early stages of the epidemic. Comprehensive blood screening, and scrupulous needle and syringe hygiene have virtually eliminated this risk in most Western countries. It remains a danger, however, in many developing countries and in parts of Eastern Europe — where blood transfusions for sick or weak infants are far more common and resources for screening blood supplies for HIV are often not available outside main hospital or laboratory centres. The USSR was the first country in the world to record infection through blood in children en masse. In 1989, hospitals in Elista, Rostov-on-Don and Volgograd recorded a total of 152 children infected from re-used needles [1].

In Romania, by May 1990 official reports registered 617 children with AIDS in a country where total recorded AIDS cases numbered only 670. The vast majority of these children were living in institutions, a situation which hampered attempts to trace their mothers: fewer than half of the mothers who were eventually found were tested and of these only 5% were HIV-positive. Since mother-to-child transmission was therefore not the main route of infection, this left contaminated blood as the principal source. The Ministry of Health has begun testing all children less than three years of age living in institutions. More than 10,500 children were tested by June 1990. Ten per cent — over 1,000 — were HIV-positive [2].

Romania has had a medical tradition of giving "microtransfusions" — 10 to 20ml of blood — to, among others, undernourished children, and malnutrition was a condition from which many of these institutionalised children suffered. One donation of contaminated blood was, therefore, enough to pass HIV to large numbers of children. Frequent cuts in gas and power supplies also meant hospitals

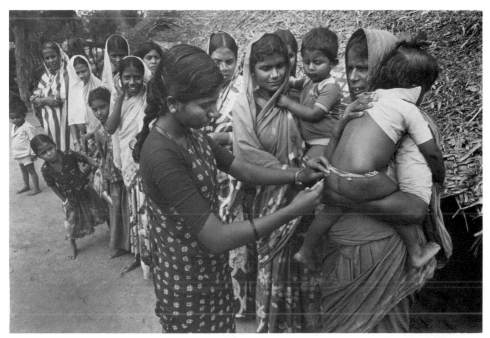

were unable to sterilise syringes and needles properly [3].

Blood transfusions do save countless lives in developing countries. They are commonly used, especially for patients suffering from malaria which annually infects nearly 300 million people, including children [4]. In many hospitals the conventional and only readily available treatment for the life-threatening anaemia, which malaria causes, has been blood transfusions.

One way of reducing risks for children is to eliminate all non-essential transfusions. To do this, some hospitals have launched intensive educational campaigns among doctors to substitute iron therapy for all but the most seriously sick children. The results are dramatic: in one hospital in Kinshasa, Zaire, the number of transfusions was reduced by almost three-quarters with no increase in deaths [5].

Early on in the course of the AIDS epidemic, doctors and health workers in developing countries worried that HIV might be inadvertently spread by re-used needles in immunisation campaigns. Yet HIV infection levels among children aged 5-14 who have been vaccinated remain very low, allaying earlier fears.

*The World Health Organization recommends that all children, whether infected with HIV or not, should receive the standard childhood vaccinations. The only exception is that children with symptoms of HIV disease should not receive the BCG vaccination against tuberculosis.*
*Ron Giling/Panos Pictures*

## DETECTING INFANT INFECTION

The parents of a baby born to an HIV-positive woman face a long and fraught period of uncertainty before they can know conclusively

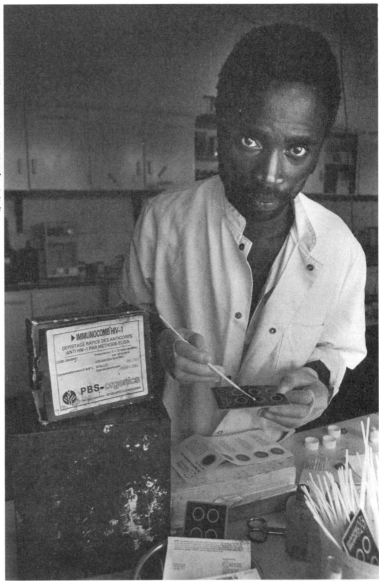

New-born babies carry their mother's antibodies to HIV for about 18 months. During that time, antibody tests cannot detect whether an infant is infected and parents face an agonising wait. Research is under way for new tests to provide earlier diagnosis, but a shortage of laboratory equipment and prohibitive costs limit the use of even standard tests in many parts of the world.
*Ron Giling/Panos Pictures*

whether their child is also infected. While children infected by contaminated blood can be diagnosed using conventional antibody tests, there is no simple and quick method of establishing whether a new-born baby whose mother is HIV-positive has contracted the virus. All babies are born with their mothers' antibodies to HIV, and conventional antibody tests do not distinguish between these and the infant's own. Only when the baby has lost the maternal antibodies — after about 18 months — is it possible to say for certain whether she or he is infected. Researchers are developing ways to detect HIV infection earlier but the methods are still too problematic and expensive to be widely used.

Because some infected babies fall ill quickly, there is often only a short time in which to start prophylactic or anti-viral treatment before AIDS develops . As more drug therapy becomes available, therefore, early diagnosis in infants will become more critical. In most parts of the developing world, however, speedy diagnosis and treatment is still largely impossible because of a shortage of testing facilities and therapeutic drugs. Often, the first indication that an infant is infected comes when he or she falls sick. For some women, a baby's illness is the first they know of their own infection.

## DISEASE PROGRESSION IN CHILDREN

Amid the uncertainty surrounding diagnosis of HIV infection in children, there is some agreement that the incubation period of HIV for children is shorter than for adults and that the earlier a child first falls ill the poorer the outcome. "Once these new-born babies develop diarrhoea — it's almost always a terminal sign," says Dr Shilalukey Ngoma, a paediatrician at Lusaka University Teaching Hospital in Zambia [6].

# Difficulties of diagnosis: Uganda

Most HIV-positive children have a long history of chronic ill-health. The mother often tells us that her child has never really been well. "He was born coughing," she will say, or "He had those swellings when he was born." Chronic diarrhoea, severely retarded growth, and recurrent fever are all common, as are skin rashes and recurrent infections. The form of malnutrition associated with HIV infection is in most cases marasmus, which gives the children a shrunken, wizened appearance.

For the most common complaints we do have the drugs available, for example, antibiotics or oral rehydration salts. We don't have gammaglobulin (an antibody compound), AZT or any other anti-viral drugs....Most of the treatment we give is on a clinical basis with little or no laboratory support.

In one family which I treated, the mother came in first with her second child. He was not growing, was always sick and treatment didn't bring any improvement. He was six months old. After a period of follow-up an AIDS diagnosis was made and the mother was found to be positive as well. By this time she was pregnant again. She delivered a baby girl without problems, who did well until she was three months old, when she too started to get sick with diarrhoea, coughing, skin rashes and swollen glands. The two children died within months of each other.

The father asked whether his children had the "new disease". He was told about all the difficulties surrounding diagnosis in children but also that it was most likely to be AIDS — the little girl had never been tested but showed all the signs. He understood his wife was infected but stopped short of asking whether he was as well. Most likely he is...

**Dr Hanne Friesen**, *currently working for a project run jointly by the AIDS Control Programme in Uganda and Save the Children Fund.*

*Some children with HIV are now surviving much longer than previously expected*

The World Health Organization has used an estimate for projection purposes that worldwide 25% of perinatally infected babies are likely to develop AIDS in the first year of life; 45% by the end of the second year; 60% by the end of the third; and 80% by the end of the fourth year [7].

Doctors agree that knowledge about HIV in children is continuously evolving, and as more data are collected, these estimates may be revised. Information from developing countries on disease progression is not readily available because follow-up studies of infected infants have generally not extended beyond two or three years. But data from the United States show that some children with HIV are now surviving much longer than previously expected.

One study suggests that there is a significant population of children who are infected but not yet diagnosed, and who may remain free of symptoms for several years. Using information about 215 children who developed AIDS by age 10, it estimated that 20% develop AIDS within the first year and 8% in each subsequent year [8]. However, the study may have slightly overestimated survival times since some children who die as a result of HIV infection are never diagnosed with AIDS. This was particularly true in the early 1980s because of the stringent diagnostic guidelines then used, which subsequently have been revised. Scientists do not yet fully understand why some infants suffer almost immediately from devastating symptoms and die very early, while others have a milder course of illness and better chances of survival.

Several studies have recorded two distinct patterns of disease progression in children who are infected by their mothers: either AIDS develops very early — within months rather than years — or the pattern is similiar to that among adults, and children stay healthy for several years without showing signs of HIV disease [9].

Many children who develop AIDS early fall sick by the age of six months, and usually before 18 months [10]. Among those who live longer, the average incubation period, while stretching over several years, is still shorter than that in adults — one study reported an average of 6.4 years, compared with an average of 10 years in adults [11]. The reason may be that an adult who becomes infected has already had to survive a barrage of different diseases or illnesses during their lifetime. When the immune system has conquered a disease once, it is then equipped to do so a second time more easily. While children do inherit some maternal antibodies which confer immunity, they do not have so extensive a "memory" in their immature immune systems as adults, so that once weakened by HIV they succumb more quickly to illness [12].

Researchers conclude, however, that as more data are collected, particularly about children who have been given anti-viral therapy and preventive treatment for infections, greater numbers of HIV-infected children will be discovered to have survived to later childhood. One recent study reported the case of a symptom-free 12-year-old US girl who had been infected at birth [13], and researchers predict that children who were originally infected before or during birth may live to be teenagers, themselves capable of sexual transmission [14].

*Children who were originally infected before or during birth may live to be teenagers, capable of passing on HIV sexually*

## TREATMENT FOR INFECTED CHILDREN

In developing countries, conventional drug therapies such as anti-fungal preparations and common antibiotics are sometimes in short supply. Health workers may lack protective clothing, disposable gloves, and sterile syringes and needles. Indeed, while North American scientists plan "high-tech" medical interventions on their young patients, including attaching portable infusion pumps which can send programmed doses of zidovudine (AZT) through their bodies, some doctors in the South struggle to provide feeding supplements, soap, disinfectant and extra bedding.

Although money still cannot buy a cure for AIDS, in the North advances in drug therapy have made it possible to postpone progression in adults from the stage of infection without symptoms to clinical AIDS. Intensive research to prolong the survival of children with AIDS is now under way.

Separate and time-consuming clinical trials of drugs have to be conducted in children and adults because young children's and babies' responses to drugs are different to those of adults and even older children. Doses have to be adjusted and drugs may not produce the same therapeutic or toxic side-effects.

"Traditionally children have not been entered into clinical trials of new drugs until the drugs have been shown to be safe and effective in adults", says Dr Anthony Fauci, associate director for AIDS research in the United States, "but we believe that the life-threatening nature of HIV infection may justify a modification of this policy....Trials of new agents are now being planned and conducted [15]." Many paediatricians are urging that drug trials for children should begin as soon as possible after initial results with adults are available.

## THE ETHICS OF EXPERIMENTAL DRUGS FOR CHILDREN

Paediatric drug experiments fuel the debate over what constitutes the best and most appropriate care for infected children. The fact that most children cannot decide for themselves whether to accept the risks and the possible pain of experimental drugs weighs heavily on those concerned. And in the case of AIDS, although parents do have to give consent, many are, of course, ill themselves. Who, then, decides: the state, foster parents, doctors?

Most regulations offering ethical guidelines on children as research subjects focus on research involving children who are already ill. Risks are weighed against the possibility of personal benefit and the promise of the discovery of more effective treatment. However, experimental treatments for infants born to HIV-positive mothers may also involve the 50-75% of children who will eventually lose their mother's antibodies and are therefore shown not to be infected. Thus they do not benefit personally from the fruits of the research.

Should research be postponed until there is a reliable means of distinguishing between the two groups? Should children of HIV-positive mothers be considered healthy or at risk of HIV infection? And what constitutes minimal risk for these children? These are just some of the questions and dilemmas doctors and parents face [16].

Best care means different things to different people. Those who advocate aggressive drug treatment for infected children cite the experience with childhood leukaemia, which 30 years ago was fatal, but which now through chemotherapy is curable in more than half of cases. "Research has to be conducted in children but you have to weigh up the pain and agony," stated a US mother whose baby son died of AIDS. "Zack received AZT just six weeks before he died. Maybe if he had gotten it sooner, it would have extended his life [17]."

Women, as mothers and formal and informal carers, are particularly involved in this difficult issue. The following chapter looks at their role in the care of HIV-infected children and adults.

# CHAPTER 6

# WHO CARES, WHO PAYS?

"The bulk of informal health care in the home is provided by women...both in the family and in the community. In practically every country, whatever its level of economic and social development, the majority of health workers are women....If the non-formal sector is also taken into account, women's contribution to health care is overwhelmingly greater than that of men," says the World Health Organization (WHO) [1].

*Without the care women provide at home, governments would face vastly increased health costs*

Without informal carers, the financial burden of formal health care in every country would be vastly increased. Home care is the key factor which allows those who are ill, disabled or old to continue to live in the community — and home care is provided mainly by women. The real cost of informal care is high. One calculation says that the value of women's work in the household alone, much of which is looking after others, if given economic value, would add an estimated one-third to the world's gross national product [2].

Worldwide, formal and informal systems of care — the hospital and the home — are mutually dependent. The question of who cares, and where, is crucial to overall costs.

## WOMEN WHO CARE

"Women's role as primary providers of health care within the family and community is usually underestimated — particularly by women themselves. They expect — and so does everybody else — that they will as a matter of course provide a range of care in the home, the workplace and the community. This they do in their roles as mothers, spouses, partners, grandmothers and sisters, and as voluntary and trained health workers," says Dr Marie-Thérèse Feuerstein, an independent consultant on health issues.

"'Care' includes attention to basic needs such as food and water, fuel for cooking and heating, and maintenance of a clean and sanitary environment. Women not only prepare and distribute food within the family, but in many countries are themselves substantial food and cash crop producers. Women are involved in childrearing practices such as breastfeeding, weaning and immunisation, and decision-making about family health care. They often provide home-based care for the disabled, convalescent and chronically sick, contributing essential

# How can you turn your back?

When the virus hit our home, we didn't run. We hung in there, and we're better people today. My own son has gone but I have mothers that call and meet with me once or twice a week. What is a mother to do? I tell them, "Hang in there, don't turn your back". You go to hospitals, you see precious, young, intelligent people lying in foetal positions. They have families, but nobody's there for them. If I'm in the hospital, I go by and I say, "I'm praying for you, I care about you". Those few little words sometimes bring back a spark of life. How can you turn your back?

In the hospital, they gave Bruce (my son) all kinds of tests, and medication which his body rejected. I'm a believer, and I trust in God, and I started praying. I asked for a little more time. I said, "Give me my child for a little while longer". And the three days that they said he would live turned into seven months.

When the doctors said there was nothing more that they could do, my family was there. The family input is very important. With Bruce not being able to talk or respond to anything, if we had not been there he wouldn't have been fed, because the nursing staff were scared. They would put the tray on the side. He couldn't talk, he couldn't do anything, but my daughter gave up her lunch hour and was there to feed and clean him. My husband always went straight from work to the hospital. I was there till my doctor stopped me because my blood pressure had shot up. I was near to a stroke, and I was forbidden to go to hospital.

I would tell them to put the phone near his ear, so that I could talk. I would let him know this was Ma. I said "I love you", but he couldn't respond. The day before his thirty-first birthday they brought him home. At that time he wasn't talking...he came home in a stupefied manner, not saying anything. I had told my grandchildren, "We're bringing Uncle Bruce home. He is not the same Uncle Bruce that you know".

After a while, by being home, within the family environment, Brucie started coming out of himself — I mean remembering, and starting to ask questions. My grandchildren said "Granma, Uncle Brucie can talk". I went into his room and he said "Hi Mom", and that was a joy. When you love somebody that inch of improvement means so much. He tried to gather his thoughts again. My grandchildren showed him how to write his name. We would bring him from the back room to the living room, and then he said he wanted his clothes back on. We waited on him like a baby. I changed diapers on a grown man just like I did when he was a baby.

Pneumonia set in and on October 22nd 1987 my son died. He was never comatose. He said "I'm tired, I need somebody to rub my back", and he put his head back on the pillow and he said he was going to dreamland. My son died with dignity.

Four months after Bruce's passing, I was beside myself, I didn't know what to do, and I walked into the Brooklyn AIDS Taskforce. I wanted to be involved in this AIDS crisis. I was going there just to answer telephones on a hotline, or something. But when the director heard my story, she said to me, "Would you be willing to go around and tell your story to somebody else?" I talked it over with my family and they said, "Do it if you feel you want to" — and I have been talking ever since. I tell people, "Don't abandon your loved ones. These are the same people who love you, that made you happy". You cannot catch AIDS by loving, caring and sharing.

I asked the Brooklyn AIDS taskforce, "Can I start a mothers' group?" I needed to start something in the minority area, where there are no big words or big money. We have mothers that come in and say, "I can't cope, I don't understand" and the first thing I tell them is, "I've been there. You can make it if you try". We close the doors, we hold hands, we cry, we hurt. We're ostracised but we're standing firm together. Bruce didn't leave me any babies, he didn't leave me any money, but he truly left me his strength [51].

**Mildred Pearson**, *United States*

elements such as affection and compassion. Some are fortunate in having access to training and supportive services. Others do not, and carry out their roles as primary carers as best they can," she adds [3].

"We in Uganda have found that when a man or a woman has HIV, if they have their own mother living then they stand a better chance. ...If they have no mother and no wife then they're in trouble," says Noerine Kaleeba, founder of The AIDS Support Organisation (TASO) in Uganda [4]. In the United States, a recent study of a random group of 275 people with AIDS found that, regardless of how HIV was transmitted, people of all racial and ethnic groups, including many gay men, received most of their unpaid care from women. Mothers were cited most often as a source of help [5].

"Many people simply go home to their parents when it is confirmed that they have HIV. Normally it is the mothers, some of whom are as old as 50 or 60, who have to care for their stricken children and see in this task a chance to provide, now more than ever, love, care and solidarity," says Jane Galvao, a Brazilian anthropologist [6].

*When a man or a woman has HIV, if their own mother is caring for them, they stand a better chance*

## FAMILY DILEMMAS — SOUTH AND NORTH

Families are the substance of communities. But the term "family" has different meanings in different cultures and societies. Whatever its composition, however, a family unit generally involves individuals who assume certain obligations to one another. In this broad sense, family-centred care is at the heart of AIDS care. In the communities worst-hit by AIDS, often more than one member of a family is affected.

### "Neglect not management"

In the context of AIDS care and prevention, the extended family network found in many developing countries is a national strength — especially where lengthy hospital care for large numbers of people is an impossibility. But it can easily be over-exploited. The UK non-governmental organisation Save the Children Fund argues that in assessing how best to allocate resources, it is vital not to overlook the coping strategies that already exist within a community but it is equally important to recognise where systems are under strain and to offer appropriate support [7].

Home care is not without cost. Elizabeth Ngugi of Nairobi University's Community Health Department has pointed out that where strong extended family kinship systems exist, the community pays willingly but dearly. Describing the care given to one young man who died of AIDS at home in Kenya, she catalogues the often

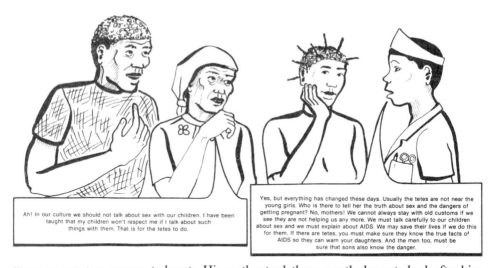

Ah! In our culture we should not talk about sex with our children. I have been taught that my children won't respect me if I talk about such things with them. That is for the tetes to do.

Yes, but everything has changed these days. Usually the tetes are not near the young girls. Who is there to tell her the truth about sex and the dangers of getting pregnant? No, mothers! We cannot always stay with old customs if we see they are not helping us any more. We must talk carefully to our children about sex and we must explain about AIDS. We may save their lives if we do this for them. If there are tetes, you must make sure they know the true facts of AIDS so they can warn your daughters. And the men too, must be sure that sons also know the danger.

**Women are on the front line of care for people with AIDS — at home, or in clinics or hospitals. Spreading information about risks — real and imagined — helps to dispel fear and prejudice.**
*"AIDS: Let us fight it together"/Women's Action Group, Harare, Zimbabwe*

uncounted costs. His mother took three months leave to look after him — with economic costs for her employer and herself; a brother took a month's leave from work to support his mother; a sister missed four weeks of high school; special food and bleach bought for cleaning bit into a limited family budget; the mother's own health deteriorated and she had to be treated, adding to the expense; and on average 10 people from the village including distant family members visited the young man daily for an average of an hour, thus a further 10 working hours were lost daily [8].

In addition, AIDS strikes hardest at the most economically productive sector of any society — men and women in their 20s, 30s, and 40s. It destroys breadwinners and leaves behind the most helpless, old and young. Within a family, grief is compounded by worries about economic survival: "The presence of a person with AIDS in an already poor family is an enormous burden. And in many of these families the person with AIDS is the breadwinner. The family are terrified at the thought of losing him or her as a person — but they also have to face losing their source of income," says Noerine Kaleeba of TASO [9].

One study suggests that when women spend long hours caring for sick family members, or when they themselves are infected and ill, the loss of labour in agriculture could have severe effects. African economies are based on rural production with agriculture accounting for at least 80% of gross domestic product and women producing most of the food eaten by their families. Food production per capita has been declining over the last 20 years [10]. With more women leaving the fields to care for sick family members, less food could be produced in some areas [11].

The capacity of the family system to provide home care is directly influenced by its access to food, work, shelter, water and basic health and social services. In many places, multiple pressures on already narrow survival margins are compounded by HIV infection. In Uganda, for example, relatives and friends in the community commonly support a bereaved family in carrying out the funeral rituals and defraying expenses. But the sheer number of AIDS deaths in some of the worst affected areas, the fact that they tend to be clustered within families, and the stigma associated with AIDS which may mean the loss of some help, all combine to undermine these normal support systems [12].

*AIDS strikes hardest at men and women in their 20s, 30s, and 40s and leaves behind the most helpless, old and young*

People with AIDS and their carers can find their lives disrupted by a devastating combination of economic and emotional pressures. A survey in Zaire showed that, compared with hospital patients without HIV, HIV-infected patients were almost twice as likely to have lost their job, to be divorced or to have moved because of their illness [13].

Some doctors and social scientists in the South are concerned that reliance on the extended family is overplayed. Without appropriate material support — such as help with basic services, training and counselling — they argue that for many people the extended family as a safety net can be no more than a myth. Health workers in Zambia insist that a reliance on home-based care which does not provide support for families, constitutes "neglect not management" [14]. The only realistic way to cope with increasing numbers of AIDS patients, they say, is to train community counsellors who will work with families providing care. A hospital-based team can then act as a back-up where necessary.

## The family and Community Care

The concept of "Community Care" has been incorporated into the welfare systems of many industrialised countries to varying degrees. It means that where possible institutionalised care is replaced or complemented by a range of health and social services to enable individuals to continue living within the community. Competition for resources, however, means that sometimes, particularly in disadvantaged areas with a high demand for services, community needs cannot always be met, and individuals may find themselves stranded without either institutional or community support.

In the North, where most HIV infection has been among gay men, the small family unit of parents and children dealing with HIV infection is often isolated for financial or social reasons within a potentially hostile community. And throughout the United States and

Europe many single mothers, unsupported by partner or extended family, are struggling to care for their sick children and themselves. Others may be dealing with their own drug abuse or that of their partner.

Jeff Montforti in San Francisco has lost two children to AIDS. He and his wife are both HIV-positive. Jeff admires the gay community in his city for "their ability to be there for one another". He adds, "I speak with many families throughout the United States and if they're not hooked up in a clinical trial...they're on their own. There are families out there now who don't have the respite that they need. ...Parents who are trying to deal with the fact that they are infected, their spouse is infected and their child is infected, don't have someone to turn to and say 'I need to take a rest — just take my kid for half an hour'. This is not there in the United States yet [15]".

The majority of families with HIV-infected children in the United States are from inner cities and on low incomes. One study of 235 children and their families found that more than 90% were living at or near the poverty line [16]. A recent US study of families where more than one person has AIDS found the medical and social care they received was "often fragmented, duplicated, episodic and unstructured" [17]. For mothers with HIV, whose babies are also infected, days can be spent running between different agencies and hospitals. A woman may miss her own appointments because of the need to care for a child or partner, or because there is no babysitter or transport. She may not even make appointments for herself at all.

"The problem I had initially was as a nurturer. Taking care of my husband [who had HIV-related illness], the household and raising a child — doing all the ordinary tasks every day — and having someone sick. Trying to meet my husband's needs and look after my child and myself — but feeling overwhelmed," says Sallie Perryman, herself HIV-positive [18].

"One-stop" clinics which coordinate medical and social services for family members with AIDS have been shown to be successful, especially for the hardest-hit families. At the Bronx-Lebanon Hospital Center in New York a model has been developed to meet the needs of a poor community, some of whom may have been at risk of infection. Pre- and post-test counselling is offered to mothers on the maternity unit. For HIV-positive mothers and babies, services are provided during the baby's regular clinic visits. Additional care or therapy is arranged through the clinic when needed. Mothers thus need fewer trips to the clinic to meet their children's and their own needs. Of the 90 children enrolled in mid-1990, 94% have not missed an appointment [19].

Many people caring for people with AIDS at home have great difficulty getting to clinics or hospitals. The most effective support services for home care are outreach programmes which bring services directly to those who need them. Home visits by doctors to supervise care provided by family or friends have been shown to reduce the number of clinic and hospital visits and the length of hospital stays [20].

At home, with appropriate care, many people who become ill from HIV infection will live for years. Many would prefer not to die in a hospital but at home surrounded by family and friends. One hospital-based multi-disciplinary home-care team in London responsible for 250 patients, during a period of 18 months enabled 30% of those terminally ill to die at home — twice the national average [21].

*An HIV diagnosis has a serious impact on the emotional stability of the whole family*

## Caring for carers

"There were so many tears and so much pain which people normally keep inside from day to day, just trying to deal with a sick child or a sick husband...", says Katie Bias describing a meeting of a group of carers for people with AIDS in the United States [22].

For informal carers, the love which binds them to the person with AIDS is often also their "Achilles heel". Caring for any child, partner, relative or friend who is going to die brings with it a huge emotional and psychological burden. Discrimination based on fear and ignorance over AIDS can cause isolation and further stress. Care-givers are often fearful of disclosing the diagnosis, which might reduce the practical and emotional support available to them [23].

Particular concerns preoccupy infected parents who also have HIV- positive children: grief over the coming loss of a child; isolation and rejection from family members and friends; feelings of guilt about infecting loved ones; and anxiety over possible future pregnancies. Many worry about who will care for the children after their own death and about any discrimination they may suffer: some children with HIV have been banned from schools and nurseries.

Parents have to deal with their own and their children's fears. They have to decide whether to tell older children that the disease is AIDS, what to tell outsiders, and whether to test children who appear healthy but may be infected.

An HIV diagnosis has a serious impact on the emotional stability of the whole family, including the brothers and sisters of a child with HIV. In one study some 43% of uninfected siblings showed behavioural problems. Girls were over-represented among this group,

*People who know someone with HIV are more likely to feel compassion for those affected by AIDS*

and researchers suggest this might be because girls were more likely than boys to be asked to help with care, particularly when the mother's illness progressed [24].

Children can be very frightened of AIDS and may be especially sensitive to stigma, adding to the psychological pressures on parents. "If he's got to be sick, why has he got to have AIDS?" asked the brother of one child with HIV. "Why can't he have cancer or something normal [25]?" "Will AIDS turn me into a monster?" asked one HIV-positive child [26].

"At first we didn't talk about me being positive," says Sallie Perryman about herself and her daughter. "Well, we talked about it with each other but I told her not to talk about it with her friends, because I worked with discrimination cases and I was afraid for her. I didn't want my diagnosis to get out into the community because I was scared for her and for me. But she had a reaction to this 'not talking' and trying to hold it in....She started showing a lot of signs of stress. Today she's coping. But the situation's put a lot of stress on her...I'm trying to relieve some of that now. She feels she has to be very responsible. She is only nine but she's a lot older than she should be for nine years old [27]."

## Familiarity breeds compassion

A Canadian study has found that, notwithstanding the general prevalence of fear and prejudice, people who know someone with HIV are more likely to feel compassion for those most affected by AIDS [28]. In the South as in the North, many prejudices have been overcome as more and more people have learnt about HIV, often through contact with someone who has been infected. Counselling HIV-positive people, their families and members of the community provides an opportunity to combat discrimination, the first step towards more general education for behaviour change.

Support groups for carers help to reduce the psychological impact of HIV infection on individuals and communities. Mothers at the "Mothers of AIDS patients" support meetings in Los Angeles are regularly joined by fathers, siblings and other relatives or friends of people with AIDS [29]. By building on shared experience, family-to-family support groups can be particularly effective. "Our counselling revolves around the family," says Noerine Kaleeba. "Once we've established a relationship with a client we want to reach out to wives, husbands, children or anyone else in the family or among friends who wants or needs to be involved as a way of supporting the individual with AIDS and each other [30]."

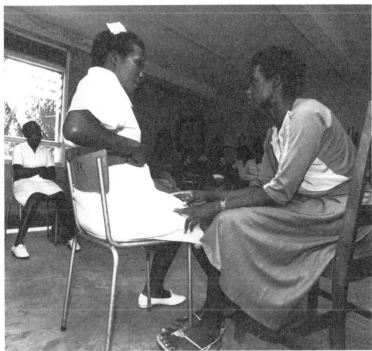

The Chikankata home-care team in Zambia learn, through role play, how to provide supportive counselling. While drug treatment can relieve some physical symptoms, understanding and compassion help to heal the isolation felt by many people with AIDS. *Carlos Guarita/ ActionAid*

## AIDS ORPHANS

The number of "AIDS orphans" — both sick and healthy children, one or both of whose parents have died from AIDS — is unknown. WHO estimate that more than 1.5 million healthy babies had been born to mothers with HIV by the end of 1989. During the 1990s, an additional 10 million uninfected children will lose one or both parents to AIDS [31].

In the developing world, where the proportion of people aged under 15 in the population is more than twice that in industrialised countries, for each adult that dies, proportionally more children are left dependent. In the South, the burden of looking after these children often falls to grandparents or other relatives, with only minimal state health, education or social services to draw upon for help. A journalist in Uganda described how she met a grandmother who was the sole adult survivor of one family and who was caring for the 12 children of her three sons, all of whom, together with their spouses, had died of AIDS [32].

Orphans with no one to care for them are still rare in the South. However, some reports suggest that people are reluctant to take on the care of children whose parents died of AIDS for fear that the children are infected [33].

# A different approach: fostering in the United States

Chelly's introduction to the foster parenthood of a "fragile" baby (a term applied to infants needing constant medical care, including infants with AIDS) began with the TV. "I was watching some news footage about what the crack [a form of cocaine] epidemic was doing to babies," she recalls. "I was shaken up by it...and...I wanted to help somehow. I had no idea how to start, so I went to my church, which sent me to a drug rehabilitation centre, which sent me to the hospital."

Chelly is not a typical foster parent in the traditional sense. As a self-employed, single woman, she would not in the past have been considered a stable caretaker for an infant, although she might have qualified to care for an older child.

As Chelly points out: "The first agency I talked to had a hard time understanding...[my] lifestyle. I had to get them to see that it would work to my advantage. My time is very flexible and I'm in a business where I can take my baby to work if I have to".

The dearth of foster parents willing to care for babies with AIDS is leading placement agencies to be more flexible. The certification process is still rigorous, but the notion of traditional nuclear families as the only appropriate setting for foster parenting has been abandoned.

"We ask a lot from them," says Lilian Johnson, assistant director of Family and Child Services of the San Francisco Social Services Department. "To take a baby and know that it's going to die, and to watch it day in and day out — that's a psychological tearing apart. Yet these foster parents are prepared to do it."

"We're finding out that 'non-traditional' people do better in this job because what we're asking is non-traditional," says Phyllis Gurdin, the social worker who founded the AIDS Foster Home Project. "We're looking for people who have had adversity in their lives and can deal with it. We don't want people changing their minds when the going gets rough. We can't have these babies abandoned all over again.

"Single women make excellent foster parents for these babies; especially nurses or someone with an elementary medical knowledge. Many of these babies are black and Hispanic, and we like to place them as close to their own cultural background as we can. We've also found that some of our best parents are gay and lesbian couples."

Chelly recalled that when she went to get Aisha from the hospital, "I realized my life was going to change forever. There were a couple of sleepless nights; I wondered what my friends and family would do. I decided to be very honest and open with them. I needed to develop a support system [but] I left the decision [to help] up to each person.

"At first some of the people who used to visit my house stopped. But others come more often because it makes them feel good to be part of Aisha's life, to be the aunts and uncles that any good family would provide. So they are a big part of the operation. I couldn't do this alone." She has also found an extended family in her church's congregation.

"You're given a certain number of days to nurture a baby", says Chelly, "so every day is important. There's a joy in that which you can't understand unless you're doing it."
**Chiori Santiago,** *United States*

For already poor families without state support the cost of care may be high. Where children are looked after by grandparents or taken into already large families, older children — particularly girls — are more likely to be needed at home to help with younger siblings and domestic chores. Uganda's national AIDS support organisation, TASO, helps foster parents to meet the additional costs, such as schoolfees, of taking on the care of orphaned children.

*The budget of the average national AIDS programme in the developing world in 1990 was less than the cost of caring for 15 people with AIDS in the US*

## Babies with no place to go

In the industrialised world, where the small family unit of parent(s) and children is more common than the extended family, orphaned babies are far more likely to be left without relatives prepared to care for them. In the United States the problem of AIDS orphans is at its most drastic in New York and New Jersey, where estimates predict that by 1995, 20,000 orphans will need permanent adoption or temporary foster care [34].

A pioneering new foster programme was established in 1985 in New York in response to the plight of "boarder babies": HIV-infected babies who remain in hospital for no medical reason but who have no home to go to. Many of these children have been placed in foster families. Some were, or are being legally adopted — overwhelmingly by their foster family. Over 90% of the foster parents recruited are still with the programme [35].

Fostering or adoption are preferable to institutional care because they are better for the babies. They are also cheaper. Babies and children of all ages respond to continuity of care. There is evidence that the mental and physical development of long-hospitalised small children, though well cared for by an ever-changing nursery staff, suffer from the lack of strong primary relationships [36].

## THE COST OF CARE

AIDS is an expensive illness. Health and social service systems the world over are already straining to meet the current needs for care, but the AIDS toll lags behind the wave of infection. Today, most HIV-positive people are still healthy but ten times more people are expected to develop AIDS in the 1990s than in the 1980s, predicts WHO.

As Jonathan Mann, former director of WHO's Global Programme on AIDS has pointed out, "nearly two-thirds of the world's AIDS cases to date and three-fourths of HIV-infected people are in developing countries. The industrialized world's total annual contribution to AIDS in the developing world is estimated at US$200 million or less; last year total expenditure for AIDS prevention and care in New York State alone was five times greater". Demand for resources is rising fastest in the countries and communities which are already the hardest hit and least able to respond. The total budget of

*Worldwide, zidovudine (AZT) remains too expensive for most people who need it*
the average national AIDS programme in the developing world in 1990 was less than the cost of caring for just 15 people with AIDS in the United States [37].

AIDS hit Africa and much of the rest of the developing world during a decade of unprecedented economic decline. During the 1980s, health spending per head dropped by over 50% in the poorest 37 countries of Africa and Latin America, and in some, infant mortality has already risen. All too often the poorest families have borne the brunt of spending cuts, rising prices and unemployment [38].

Inequity is growing within as well as between countries. With many governments worldwide struggling to find funds for health care, concerns have been raised about the allocation of resources. Globally, AIDS is viewed as more of an urban disease than a rural one. Does this attitude threaten to direct funds yet again into high-tech hospitals and medicine because so many young urban adults are affected?

In the United States in March 1990, following extensive clinical trials, the regulatory Food and Drug Administration extended the licence for the use of zidovudine (AZT) to symptom-free people whose immune systems are nonetheless damaged by HIV. Although contested by some scientists, the rationale is that the drug can limit the progression of disease at this early stage. According to these guidelines, half of all HIV-positive people in the United States could theoretically be offered zidovudine — a potential 10-fold increase in the use of the drug — with enormous implications for cost and resources[39]. In 1989, the estimated annual cost of zidovudine therapy in the United States was calculated at US$5 billion [40].

Zidovudine is an extremely beneficial treatment but many of those hit by AIDS are too poor to buy the drug. In the United States "...there are some 35 million people without health insurance of any kind, most of them in poorly paying jobs that don't provide insurance. Millions more possess only skimpy insurance. These two groups constitute a population that tends to receive little or no care at all," says US commentator Dan Greenberg [41].

In developing countries the idea of "early intervention" with drugs to delay the progression of HIV disease is even more meaningless. Worldwide, zidovudine remains too expensive for most people who need it.

At the same time, US researchers have looked at the care provided for people with AIDS in hospital and found that stays are often longer than necessary. Discharge from hospital is often delayed because of difficulties in coordinating out-of-hospital care [42]. Daily hospital costs represent the largest chunk of direct spending on treatment for people with AIDS, say US and Mexican researchers. Fewer and shorter hospital stays could lead to dramatic savings in overall costs [43].

In the United States, children with AIDS are hospitalised more often than adults and at a higher cost [44], three times higher, according to one study [45]. This is because children suffer from more infections and often cannot be discharged because their parents have died or are too sick to care for them at home. At New York's Harlem Hospital, over 20% of paediatric AIDS costs and one-third of the total in-patient days result from social rather than medical factors [46].

Hospital treatment can be replaced with out-patient treatment only if additional care is available at home — which frequently means from women.

"In the South, Primary Health Care programmes have made use of women's traditional multi-faceted role as primary care providers. Child health strategies, for example, stress the education of mothers in improving weaning practices. Illiterate grandmothers are trained in safer birth techniques and sisters are taught to give basic physiotherapy to disabled siblings. It will be necessary to increase the range and sustainability of community responses to support this caring — and to ensure that the costs paid by women are recognised and supported," says Dr Marie-Thérèse Feuerstein, a health consultant.

"The problem, however," she continues, "is that primary health care itself is reeling under the impact of economic recession. Existing health and social infrastructures in many areas remain very centralised, preventing a flexible response to locally defined needs. In some places, increasing moves to 'privatise and commercialise' run counter to the types of policies and actions needed to combat the AIDS pandemic. In addition, much of situation analysis, policy-making, action, and monitoring in the field of AIDS prevention and control tend to reflect Western concepts and are implemented by organisations of largely male membership. This handicaps the fuller and more equal involvement of women [47]."

*Genuine community care may be the best means of spreading accurate information about HIV*

## A NEW PARTNERSHIP: HEALTH WORKERS AND FAMILY CARERS

"Any attempt to prevent the spread of HIV and to care for those who are infected must involve people from many different disciplines, working at different levels — teachers, parents, health and social workers, traditional healers, birth attendants — plus families and communities," says school teacher Fernanda Ramos, a founder member of the Senagalese branch of the Society for Women and AIDS in Africa (SWAA) [48].

*Over-isolation of infected individuals fuels stigmatisation*    Genuine community care for people with AIDS is arguably the best means available of spreading accurate information about HIV infection, and encouraging people to protect themselves by their own behaviour. Over-isolation of infected individuals fuels stigmatisation and encourages other people to feel themselves immune from risk.

Suggestions for changes in health care practices to cope with the AIDS pandemic are part of the broader movement for change which inspired the ideals of Primary Health Care in the South and Community Care in the North in the late 1970s and 80s. Essentially both rely upon a critical shift in the relationship between health care and other service providers and family carers. The underlying principle, as Susan Rifkin and Gill Walt at the London School of Hygiene and Tropical Medicine point out, is "not merely health service improvements. It is understanding the range of social, political and economic factors which ultimately influence the improvement of health" [49].

In communities all over the world, grassroots organisations responded before governments to the often desperate needs for AIDS prevention and care. And people with HIV infection chose to participate in the processes of prevention, care and research. Many of the traditional roles of service providers and recipients — the doctor-patient relationship — have  been radically called into question. It is essential that home care-givers are included in discussions and decisions, and acknowledged for the expertise they have acquired through living with someone with AIDS, say US researchers [50].

The AIDS pandemic has shown just how far most societies are from realising the principles of Primary Health Care and Community Care. Valuing and investing in available family and community resources may be the expressed intention but the reality is more often official neglect and exploitation of society's unpaid carers, who are mostly women. Only a deliberate reallocation of resources which acknowledges and supports home and community care can spread the burden more evenly.

# CHAPTER 7

# AIDS PREVENTION AND THE STATUS OF WOMEN

"The time has come not just to say 'no' to unwanted sex, or unprotected sex, or unwanted conception — it is time to say 'no' to inequality, to discrimination and to lack of choices. It is...necessary to be bold....As a result of AIDS, in many societies, teaching and dialogue about sexuality has been permitted for the first time. This dialogue must be used to broaden awareness and discussion of gender roles and the social and economic dimensions of what it means to insist on use of a condom, or to say 'no'," said Jonathan Mann, former director of the World Health Organization's (WHO) Global Programme on AIDS, speaking at the First International Conference on the implications of AIDS for mothers and children in 1989 [1].

As the heterosexual spread of HIV increases, the relationship between social and economic advantage and risk behaviour is becoming clearer [2]. The equation is not new. The poor and disadvantaged are known to suffer more from many avoidable health risks and their ranks are increasingly made up of women. "The feminisation of poverty is increasingly typical of both richer and poorer countries....In the United States, one of the most prosperous countries on earth, two out of three adults living below the poverty level in 1983 were women....But among all those who live in poverty, women who are the rural poor of the Third World are the most disadvantaged [3]." The burden of HIV infection falls most heavily on the poorest women in the poorest communities around the world. The implications of the changing pattern of the epidemic are considerable.

In 1990, at the end of the first decade of the AIDS pandemic, most of the concrete evidence of behaviour change comes from statistics in the United States and Europe showing that homosexual men are adopting safer sex. While the world still has a great deal to learn from these successes, repeating them in the wider heterosexual community and in the South may be much more difficult.

The US homosexual community which pioneered AIDS education is in many ways unique. Although marginalised, it is equipped with other advantages. It is a fundamentally cohesive group with high levels of education and employment. It had already confronted prejudice prior to AIDS, and thus had developed an organised, politicised network accustomed to lobbying and campaigning, with access to media and money. It was able to draw on thousands of

*Some of the* volunteers for whom AIDS was a high priority.
*most powerful*    In the North, many of the women affected by AIDS as individuals,
*educators are* mothers and carers are black and Latina. Research undertaken in New
*proving to be* York City among AIDS service organisations in their communities
*women with* suggests they have far fewer resources to commit to network building
*HIV or AIDS* or lobbying [4]. Most of their time and money has to be devoted to the
direct provision of services. Women in developing countries have
fewer resources still.

## PARTICIPATION

"Policy has both a process and a content: has the process involved
women — those most directly affected by the policies?" asked
Jonathan Mann in 1989 [5]. Unless women participate in senior level
policy-making bodies, research and education focusing on their needs
will continue to be under-resourced.

Globally, relatively little attention is paid to medical and
behavioural research into HIV issues as they specifically affect
women, for example, the effects of zidovudine (AZT) in women and
children or female-controlled HIV prevention methods. Nor are
sufficient resources directed towards education programmes designed
specifically for women. There is an obvious parallel with development
strategies since the 1960s where women's role in the development
process was initially largely ignored by those responsible for the
planning, design and implementation of programmes [6].

Women's organisations and those concerned with the impact of
AIDS on women are calling for more resources. "In the history of
development initiatives, women have often been educated to change
a familiar behaviour, but too often have not been provided with the
necessary tools and services to facilitate that change," says Chloe
O'Gara of the US organisation AIDSCOM [7]. Having more power to
make decisions on the allocation of resources is a vital first step,
argues Marge Berer of the Women's Global Network for
Reproductive Rights. Women's choices and priorities must find
public voice among policy-makers. "If women do not speak up and
act for their own empowerment, whether in the economic arena, the
environment movement, or in education, health or housing, our
interests will be forgotten or conveniently subsumed under those of
men," she warns [8].

## COMMUNICATION: WOMAN TO WOMAN

Spreading the word about how women can protect themselves from
HIV has become a goal for women educators from all walks of life

and in communities the world over.

Some of the most powerful spokeswomen are proving to be women with HIV or AIDS. Their involvement dramatically increases the emotional impact of the information provided [9]. "During presentations we see the shock on people's faces when they realise that we're not three-headed monsters, and in fact our lifestyles are very similar to theirs," says Sheila Gilchrist of the UK-based organisation Positively Women. "The stigma of AIDS means some people perceive us to be a race of people apart; and we're not. Our needs are the same as anyone else: we need a roof over our heads, food in our stomachs, and a degree of stability in our lives. We're just mothers bringing up our children in the best way we can [10]."

*We see the shock on people's faces when they realise that we're not three-headed monsters*

AIDS educators and counsellors must talk the same language as their intended audience. "Targeting the right kinds of information for the right groups of people has got to be the bottom line," says Katie Bias, herself HIV-positive and doing HIV education work with the Women's Outreach Network of the US National Haemophilia Foundation. "The information has to be culturally appropriate, which means going to the experts — the people who know the community. Literature and videos have to be tailored to needs...we have to put aside the taboos we have about what can and can't be discussed...we just have to get the word out any way we can, and if it means using words society doesn't find acceptable — well, it's either that or a continuing and increasing spread of disease [11]."

To be effective within any community, education messages must come from trusted representatives. "Support has to come from within the community," says Sallie Perryman of New York's AIDS Institute, born and raised in Brooklyn, a predominantly black area of the city. "There is a track record of distrust because...nothing has ever been done in our communities — in terms of the quality of medical care and provision — from the outside. What has to happen is that our community has to attack the problem and then get assistance from outside. We need external resources but they have to come through people who speak the right language....First you've got to get past the trust issues [12]."

The possibility of behaviour change relies on educators offering positive, realistic and sustainable alternatives to existing patterns of behaviour. Those most likely to fulfil these criteria are people who are talking to their equals: peer group educators. "Group experiences and subsequent peer education training has resulted in women becoming public speakers who had never considered such activity before," say researchers [13].

Street outreach — delivering information to people in the

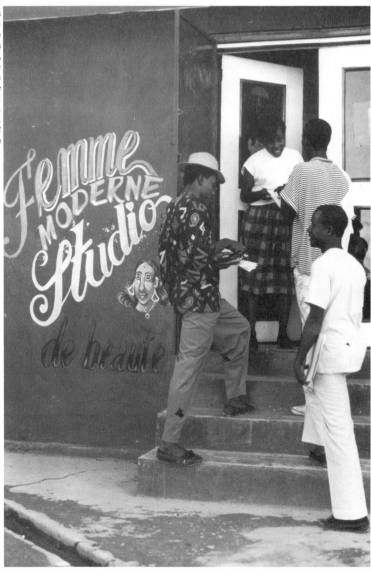

AIDS education, if it is to succeed, has to be innovative about where and when to reach its audience. In Haiti, health promotors have found Port-au-Prince's beauty parlours are effective condom and AIDS information outlets for the city. *Hilary Hughes/AIDS Action*

neighbourhoods where they live and work — is a labour-intensive part of many women's AIDS education programmes worldwide. In Brooklyn, New York, the Association for Drug Abuse Prevention and Treatment (ADAPT) runs a street outreach project in areas with high rates of drug use. Support groups and a drop-in centre also provide settings where women feel able to talk freely. Most of the women ADAPT reaches are aged between 16 and 25, and Latina or black. The majority work as prostitutes and many inject drugs, as do their clients. ADAPT workers offer the women condoms, literature about AIDS and needle-sterilising kits. If women request it, staff will try to get them into drug treatment programmes or out of prostitution, but the main thrust of the programme is risk reduction [14].

In Haiti, the community-based Haitian Centre for Social Services is working through hundreds of the brightly painted beauty parlours scattered throughout the poor neighbourhoods of the capital Port-au-Prince. The proprietors have become effective AIDS educators, handing out leaflets and condoms and discussing AIDS with their customers — reaching some three-quarters of the women in the city [15].

Finding out which issues touch women most deeply is crucial. "Sometimes the women that we visit don't seem very interested in the subject of AIDS. It seems remote to them, unconnected to their lives, but they change immediately when we mention the dangers that their children face," says Professor Lourdes Arguelles who heads the Women's Peer Education Programme in Long Beach, California. One of the videos used by the programme has as its principal character a Guatemalan woman whose son has HIV. The woman's personal story has a more powerful impact on the audience than any recitation of AIDS statistics [16].

## Networks

A number of new networks or coalitions have been established specifically to address the issues that AIDS raises for women. The Society for Women and AIDS in Africa (SWAA), a continent-wide organisation, was founded in 1988. "Professional African women decided to take action in providing leadership based on a clear understanding of the strong effective role that they are determined to play as scientists, wives, mothers, sisters, community leaders and policy-makers who are committed to improving the health care and social conditions of women. This will be done from a woman's perspective, and particularly taking into consideration the different deeply-rooted cultural beliefs and practices of African societies and the socio-economic realities and needs of the African woman [17]." SWAA now has national branches in 15 countries across Africa.

AIDS awareness programmes can also be built into existing networks and services. In the United States, for example, women who may be more vulnerable to HIV infection include teenagers, drug users, and their partners — all of whom are known to be difficult to reach through traditional health education systems. But such women are seen regularly by staff in family planning and drug abuse clinics and by other medical and social service personnel. The US Women's AIDS Network recommends providing training and support to this

*There is a* diverse range of workers, so that they can become AIDS educators to
*renewed* the women they already serve.
*urgency for*     Religious institutions can also provide networks which reach
*increased male* women. In groups which undertake pastoral work related to health,
*participation* women and children, the leadership is usually female and there is a
*in* high level of trust. In Brazil, for example, a recent poll found that 80%
*contraception* of the population regard the church as the most trusted of official
institutions [18].

Existing women's organisations are also taking up the AIDS
challenge. Often their experience in dealing with sensitive areas in the
past points a way forward for dealing with AIDS. In Zimbabwe, the
Harare Women's Action Group (WAG) interviewed women and men
in cities and rural areas to assess their concerns about AIDS. After
discussing their findings with doctors and sociologists, they designed
a cartoon book, "AIDS: Let us fight it together". The style is
down-to-earth and accessible using characters of different ages and
backgrounds with whom readers can identify easily.

## Family planning

Family planning and maternal and child health networks are a prime
route for reaching women. But they still have a long way to go, for
millions of women have only minimal access to any form of
contraceptive advice or products.

The hazards are clear. Half a million women each year die from
the effects of too frequent pregnancies coupled with poor health care
— a death toll equivalent to a jumbo jet crashing every four hours,
every day, with no survivors [19]. Most of the "passengers" are from
the South: 99% of maternal deaths are in developing countries,
concentrated among the poorest women. In countries where safe
abortions are unobtainable, an estimated 200,000 women die each
year of illegal abortions; millions more are permanently injured due
to their attempts to limit the number of theirchildren [20].

In addition to arguing for better contraceptive advice and
technology, including the female condom, many women also point
out that efforts are needed to educate men to their responsibilities.
Family planners in the North, even in the pre-AIDS world, were
raising concerns that young men particularly were abdicating any
form of responsibility for sexual relations: "the price paid for the
benefit of contraceptive autonomy offered by the Pill to young women
was an increasing indifference by male partners to making responsible
preparation for sexual relations...", comments Philip Meredith of the
International Planned Parenthood Federation (IPPF). "By the time of

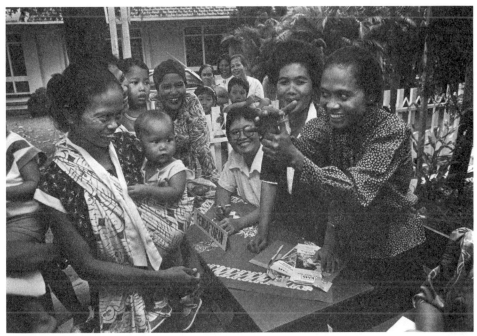

the initial health scares of the contraceptive wonder-drug in the mid-1970s, it was no longer so easy to persuade the male generation to take back the share of contracepting which they had once held when methods were restricted to the condom and diaphragm," he adds.

Getting down to basics: condom promotion and family planning advice in the right hands can break down barriers and provoke open discussion and laughter.
*Ron Giling/Panos Pictures*

The argument that male involvement should be increased has its opponents. "Many women...particularly in the developing world would be apprehensive at the prospect of the family planning movement encouraging a partial shift of emphasis to increase male involvement in fertility control," acknowledges Meredith. "The history of women's fight to control their fertility through contraceptive use is a relatively short one, and this fight was in no small part aimed to diminish the authoritarian control exercised by male partners and male community leaders, health professionals, etc," Meredith adds [21]. With the spread of HIV, and without as yet a female-controlled barrier method of protection, the need for male participation in contraception has a renewed urgency.

Routine gynaecological care provided by local doctors could also provide an opportunity to reach women with information on AIDS and STD prevention and care. Dutch doctor Marge Meijer tells how many women only reveal what may be symptoms of STDs when asked specifically about abdominal pain, discharge or discomfort during sex. This "gentle encouragement" is crucial since "often women will get used to these conditions and put up with them because they are too embarrassed to mention them to their doctor". Some 70% of her patients with sexually transmitted diseases (STDs) are women, most under 30. She feels strongly that doctors should take the opportunity to provide information about the long-term consequences of unsafe sex, particularly the threat to fertility. The desire to protect fertility can be a powerful motivator for women to practice safer sex [22].

# Reaching women and men through family planning networks

It is always said that family planners have the necessary skills to carry out AIDS prevention. Experience has shown, however, that a new direction is needed if family planning programmes are to help clients to practise safer sex as a routine part of their work rather than making it a separate programme.

Talking about AIDS to clients requires talking about sexual relationships, numbers of partners and types of sexual practice, all of which may be viewed by worker and client as an invasion of privacy, embarrassing, threatening, time-consuming and at the end of the day, achieving little.

Furthermore, although joint responsibility and communication between couples about family planning has always been encouraged, many women obtain a female method, such as the Pill, at the clinic without their partners being involved or even aware of it. Often workers concerned about women's rights would rather keep it that way, seeing the clinic as a place where women have autonomy over their bodies. They may also have a certain amount of discomfort at the thought of examining and counselling the unfamiliar male.

This situation will have to change, at least until female barrier methods become available, because the condom is a male method and men are usually aware that they are using it. Family planners need training which will help them to counsel men and couples and to work with groups of men of all ages as well as women. Unless men are treated as responsible, caring human beings rather than irresponsible children who have to be seduced or cajoled into good behaviour, the promotion of safer sex is unlikely to make much impact.

Family planning programmes can also broaden their services to include the early detection and treatment of all STDs through appropriate sexual history taking, and screening. Women are frequently happier to get an STD check at the Family Planning Association (FPA), than at the local out-patient department, often simply because they are more likely to be examined by a woman. An emphasis on the protection of fertility and maternal and child health can take away any potential stigma attached to AIDS involvement, and improve the image of the FPA as an organisation concerned with family health rather than "birth control".

**Gill Gordon**, *communications and education advisor, AIDS Unit, International Planned Parenthood Federation, United Kingdom*

## STRATEGIES FOR CHANGE:
## CONTROL VERSUS EMPOWERMENT

At the beginning of the 1990s, evidence of women changing their *Safer sex is* sexual behaviour to protect themselves against HIV is slight. One area *the only option* where positive examples of change in response to information can be *for women sex* found is among female sex workers. As with the experience of the *workers* homosexual community, there are lessons to be shared. Perhaps the key debate is over the relative merits of regulation and control versus empowerment as motivators for change.

Women in the sex industry have attracted considerable attention as a result of the AIDS pandemic. In the first instance, concern over their position in the human chain of HIV infection is logical. Everyone who has unprotected sex with a number of partners is at risk of HIV infection and needs to be able to protect himself or herself and partners. Scientists tracking the path of HIV are aware that people who have high rates of partner change and who practise unprotected sex have a disproportionate impact on the spread of HIV.

Yet, as prostitutes' organisations point out, the issues of safer sex are the same for them as for anyone, since it is not prostitution itself but behaviour which determines risk. Cheryl Overs of the Victoria Prostitutes' Collective in Australia argues that "safer sex is the only option for women sex workers like everyone else. Why should they be singled out for a sex ban, when other people at risk of transmitting the virus aren't? The fact that money changes hands is neither here nor there. The virus doesn't travel on dollar bills...[23]".

The logic of such arguments, however, is often lost in deep-rooted and emotional attitudes to prostitution, and to female sexuality generally; attitudes which are revealed in the kind of language used, according to Priscilla Alexander, former co-director of COYOTE, the US National Task Force on Prostitution . "Prostitutes are too rarely described in the scientific literature as women who need services because of their 'illnesses', rather they are described as 'reservoirs of infection,' 'pools of disease,' and 'the single most important factor in HIV transmission'. In contrast, the wives of men who are infected with HIV have been described as 'cul-de-sacs'....Because prostitutes are seen as the 'source of contagion', and not 'recipients'...discussions of how to reduce the spread of HIV infection emphasise the clients' risks and their convenience first," she adds [24].With or without the threat of HIV, it is this perception of prostitutes as dangerous women which provides the rationale for policies of discrimination, regulation and even imprisonment. But where women sex workers have taken steps to protect themselves (and hence their clients and partners) from HIV, the change has relied upon empowerment rather than control.

## Prostitute power

*The virus doesn't travel on dollar bills* Education projects run by and with women sex workers provide some of the best examples of programmes which support behaviour change by encouraging women to take on leadership roles, and where access to information has led to effective action.

The Prostitutes' Collective of Victoria in Australia conducts many programmes aimed at integrating AIDS-prevention knowledge into all aspects of the diverse and recently legalised sex industry. Among their innovative activities is a "hello sailor" campaign which provides AIDS education for visiting servicemen [25]. And in Amsterdam, the Netherlands, the prostitutes' rights group De Rode Draad (The Red Thread) has conducted a humorous campaign for sex workers and clients using a sticker which says " Ik Doe Het Met" — I do it with (a condom). The stickers have been placed in toilets of bars and discos and some women put them in their windows to inform potential clients.

Despite difficulties over the use, availability and cost of condoms for women sex workers, some programmes report dramatic increases in condom use — and consequent decreases in new HIV infections.

In Nigeria, a number of projects with prostitutes have been set up in an attempt to pre-empt widespread infection. In Borno State in Nigeria during 1987-88, more than 1,000 women prostitutes benefited from health education and counselling after being tested for HIV. A large number of this group took up routine condom use. A follow-up study in 1989 showed HIV infection rates of 1.6% for those who had been involved in the awareness programme compared with 6.1% among women who had not been counselled [26].

In Accra, Ghana, in 1987, selected sex workers within a particular community were taught about condom use and supplied with free condoms to distribute to others. About 6% of the women had tested positive, and although many had heard about AIDS their information was not always accurate. Two years later, clients who refused to use condoms faced a clear choice — they were being told to wear them or go away, since in the words of Alice, chairperson of a prostitutes' association, "we can't risk getting this disease just for money " [27].

According to Ghanaian AIDS expert Dr Alfred Neequaye, many of the poorest prostitute women "see themselves as victims of an unjust society, first as a result of underdevelopment, and second because of the traditional discrimination against women...most see themselves as doing a job to make a living, but would obviously be quite happy if they could get alternative employment [28]". Some projects, recognising this, aim to introduce income-generating activities as a long-term alternative to prostitution, in parallel with education campaigns and condom distribution.

## Regulation and control

The public health consequences of identifying the risk of HIV infection with prostitutes could be enormous, say women's groups and AIDS workers. Stigmatisation of prostitutes as causers and carriers of HIV implicitly allows everyone else off the risk hook and leads to measures designed to protect clients, not the women themselves [29]. In 1988, participants at a WHO consultation on the prevention and control of STDs among prostitutes and their clients criticised compulsory HIV screening of prostitutes and the distribution of "cards indicating a non-infected status". Such measures "impede the application of effective prevention measures" by encouraging male clients, who may carry the virus, to refuse to use condoms because they think they are not at risk — thus putting the women at risk. Nor is screening foolproof: recently infected people may not produce antibodies to the virus for several months. The consultation also warned that attempts to prohibit prostitution by law without offering retraining and other employment options were destined to fail, and that repressive measures could drive prostitution underground, hampering AIDS prevention programmes [30].

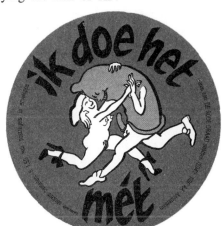

*"I do it with" (a condom): a window sticker used by Dutch prostitutes alerts clients in advance.*
*De Rode Draad, Amsterdam, the Netherlands*

Furthermore, some women have no choice but to continue working. A study of Filipina prostitutes showed that some HIV-positive prostitutes continued to work for several months after their official permits were revoked. Researchers concluded that counselling and training for other jobs are most effective in changing behaviour [31].

The first decade of the AIDS pandemic has seen conflict, imprisonment and court cases as a result of attempts to police sex workers. "Thirteen US states require anyone convicted or charged with prostitution to be tested for antibodies to HIV. Sweden, Germany and Australia have quarantined some women who continued to work as prostitutes after learning they were HIV-positive," reports US AIDS worker Priscilla Alexander. In India, HIV-positive prostitutes have been detained, sometimes for several years. And in Thailand,

*Some of the most successful examples of changes to safer practices are to be found among women sex workers*

# Prostitution: providing an alternative

In Kaolack, Senegal, a group of more than 200 part- and full-time prostitutes are involved in a programme designed first to improve their quality of life and ultimately to enable them to make an alternative living to prostitution. Twenty eight per cent of the women are infected with HIV compared with a rate of 0.5% found by some studies among the population at large in Senegal.

Most of the women live and work in rooms just large enough for them and a client. There is never more than a couple of inches of water in the bottom of a bucket for washing each day; rotting rubbish in the area outside is a permanent problem; malaria and other diseases are common. At about US$1 per client, survival is a constant struggle. Eighty per cent of the women are divorced and many have children to support.

The first stage of the project provides the women and their children with primary health care facilities and social and psychological support. Staff provide advice on health and sex education and nutrition and a range of services including pre- and post-natal care and immunisation.

When provided with condoms for use with clients, the women were quick to express their enthusiasm. Building on improvements in physical and mental health, the second phase of the project will include training for co-operative income-generating activities — laundry and sewing services, peanut-butter manufacture — as alternatives to prostitution [54].

"AIDS-free" cards have been distributed to sex workers who test negative. Those who test positive lose their jobs and are sent home to their villages, but are replaced by other young women in search of an income. "What are they going to do when they get to the last woman?" asks Chantawipa Apisook of the Thai organisation Empower. She argues that in effect the government uses its policy of testing women in the sex industry "to say that Thailand can offer AIDS-free women" to international sex tourists [32].

## Youth education

It is much easier, say AIDS educators, to teach safer sexual practices, including condom use, to young people who have not yet developed unsafe practices. Reaching boys and girls together also provides a chance to discuss gender roles before they influence sexual decision-making. "Children need to learn the facts about AIDS — the younger the better, and they should be instilled with a sense of self-worth and self-respect. Instead of stressing that marriage is a woman's only goal in life, I'd like to see parents of young daughters emphasise the importance of their future financial and emotional independence as well. Then young women may feel less pressure to engage in unsafe behaviour," says UK AIDS worker Sheila Gilchrist [33].

Much can be learned for HIV education strategies from the

# "Education, not discrimination": A court case in India

A court in Madras, India, in July 1990 ordered the release of five prostitutes, originally arrested for prostitution in 1985. A chance test by a researcher on blood samples taken from one woman at the detention centre showed she had antibodies to HIV. Subsequently, other detainees tested positive. On the basis of these results, the women, who completed their sentences in 1987, were refused release.

In November 1989, the Public Prosecutor of the Madras High Court was notified of the illegal nature of such a detention. After four months with no action, a writ of habeas corpus seeking the release of five of the women was filed. The court action sought to highlight the fact that the policy of isolation was not only discriminatory but also an ineffective response to the spread of HIV which could have harmful repercussions.

The petition argued, among other things, that the detention grossly violated the constitutional rights of the women; that the blood tests on the women were done without precautions to protect their confidentiality; that no attempts had been made to isolate people who were HIV-positive other than prostitutes: and that there was gender discrimination because for every HIV-positive woman, at least one HIV-positive man was free, able to infect other women.

The court appointed an advocate commissioner to enquire into the matter. She reported that the women were being held against their will, and that despite being inmates of the centre for five years, they remained ignorant of the facts about HIV. The court concluded that the detention was illegal and ordered the women's release.

The case attracted particular attention because the previous month, 854 Bombay prostitutes had been "rescued" by a voluntary organisation and brought to Madras, to be returned to their families. Six hundred and forty of the women were then tested for HIV, of whom 454 had positive results. They were immediately confined to remand homes.

Days after the July verdict on the original five women, all illegally detained prostitutes in Madras, including the 454 "Bombay women", were freed.

Reactions to the case have been mixed. One top official, who requested anonymity, admitted that the order was "a relief". "We were finding it difficult to hold so many women. ...Personally I don't think holding them will help and I'm glad to let them go." Around the country a number of lawyers and doctors as well as women's organisations have welcomed the judgment.

Others hold a different opinion. "What's the use of releasing them when you know they will infect so many others? It's irresponsible," said one prominent social worker in Madras.

Some of the women have no option but to return to prostitution. Though efforts were made to educate them on HIV and AIDS — and their own status as carriers — before their release, it is unlikely that many will use condoms with future clients. They are often powerless to do so and their clients and pimps, like most of the general population, are ignorant about HIV prevention. The Chairman of the Social Welfare Board, recognising this, argues that there is an urgent need for a rehabilitation plan. "It's not fair that the women be left to fend for themselves. Long-term detention...is unrealistic. And as the numbers of HIV-positive people swell, it seems inescapable that public education, not discrimination, is the answer."

**Shyamala Nataraj,** *India*

A sex education booklet for Native Americans goes to heart of the matter. Rather than telling young people what they should do, it provides information. Above all, it encourages a sense of self-esteem in teenage women so that they can make their own decisions.
*Native American Women's Health Centre, South Dakota, US*

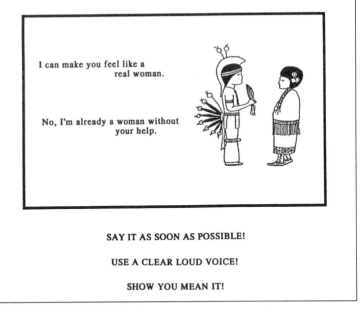

SAY IT AS SOON AS POSSIBLE!

USE A CLEAR LOUD VOICE!

SHOW YOU MEAN IT!

approaches of teenage STD and pregnancy prevention programmes. Access to information and services, skills training, and enhanced self-esteem are all excellent motivators for young people to use contraceptives or delay intercourse. Once again, the lesson seems to be that empowerment is a more effective approach than regulation or control.

Yet there has always been tension between parents and others who feel too much information — particularly for young women — is dangerous, and those who believe too little knowledge is more so. In many cultures, women "grow up being 'protected' from sexual knowledge in the traditional sense...sexuality is often viewed as polluting," says US anthropologist Professor Vincent Gil [34]. The threat of AIDS has made the debate simultaneously more controversial and more urgent. In the United States, for example, opinion polls in the late 1980s showed that 94% of parents believe that schools should develop AIDS education programmes. At the same time many parents worry that AIDS and sexuality education promotes or encourages early sexual experimentation. They also fear that schools might present views that run counter to their values [35].

Research indicates that sex education in schools does not appear to encourage teenagers to initiate sexual activity, and may increase the likelihood of them using contraception if they are having sex [36]. Similarly, when sex is discussed in the home, teenagers are less likely to begin sexual activity early and more likely to use contraception when they do, say researchers [37]. "Traditionally, the world over, we have always shied away from talking about sex and our children have just discovered things by accident," says Noerine Kaleeba, director of TASO the Ugandan AIDS care organisation. "Now we have to change. It costs us more not to than it does to speak about sex, but it must be in such a manner that it is not going to turn our children away from sex completely, but will give them the facts they need to protect themselves. This must be done at all levels but particularly in schools and within the family, tailored towards the understanding and the needs of children at different ages. Women must talk to their children — both sexes," she asserts [38].

*Children need to learn the facts about AIDS — the younger the better*

Mary Amanyire Byangire, a Ugandan social worker, shares her sense of urgency: "In our community, you grow up with mother looking after you but she may not tell you anything about how to have a boyfriend or anything else. They usually leave it for you to find out for yourself. But it's high time we realised that this cannot work in the present situation with AIDS. We must educate our young girls, our young ones — we should stop being ashamed — before it's too late [39]". Uganda's President Museveni, as well as personally appealing to young people to refrain from having more than one sex partner, has called on all parents to reduce the 'bride price' which must be found before marriage. If the sum to be exchanged between families before marriage is too high, young people may have to wait a long time before getting married. "The slogan here is 'Love Carefully and Stick to One Partner'. How can one do that when one has no partner due to high cost!" says Miria Matembe, chairperson of Action for Development [40].

The vital role of peer education is a tenet of most programmes which aim to limit the spread of HIV through a change in behaviour and peer pressure is never more powerful than during adolescence. While parents and teachers have a major role to play in AIDS education, materials presented by other young people or which appeal to peer-group loyalties are proving more effective than warnings delivered by adults. This approach has been successfully developed by, for example, US high school students who run a free AIDS telephone hotline; by secondary school boys in Zambia who have set up anti-AIDS clubs pledging chastity before marriage; and by street children in the Dominican Republic who are extending their street hawking to include selling condoms.

Mexico's family planning association, MEXFAM, bases its philosophy on the recognition that young people should be given the information and help to make responsible decisions about sex for themselves, instead of following the conventional approach in which they are told what they should think and do. Hence MEXFAM's youth

# Mexico's youth involvement programme

Working on the basis that most young people's sexual relations are spontaneous and irregular, Mexico's family planning association, MEXFAM, aimed to create a community-based 'movement', run by and for the young. The programme is targeted at people between the ages of 10-20 living in low-income areas. Contraceptives are available through volunteers, without the need to visit a clinic.

The starting point of the programme is research into the needs of the young community and the establishment of contacts in schools, youth clubs, gangs and places of work. While MEXFAM staff provide the initial training and policy direction, daily programme planning is very much the responsibility of the supervising MEXFAM coordinator and his or her team of young promoters.

All promoters are volunteers: students or unemployed adolescents with an interest in social work, psychology, nursing, etc, who wish to do community work which will help them gain experience and increase their chances of employment.

The principal incentives for young people to become promoters include gaining access to MEXFAM facilities, the status they acquire within the community through training, and not least the small profit they are allowed to make from the sale of contraceptives. The family planning organisation provides supplies to promoters at a small charge, which they then sell at an agreed price. The difference is theirs. Opposition to the idea of condom distribution is rare in Mexico, partly because of the well-understood reality of sex among teenagers, and also because of the fear of AIDS.

The programme depends heavily on creating links between parents, school teachers and youth, with school teachers being encouraged to become "volunteer coordinators". Educational materials, particularly video films, talk about condoms and their use, but look also at family relations, particularly between parents and children. The traditional "machismo" culture of Mexico places a heavy burden on young men who are forming their first relations with girlfriends. So many young people experience an unplanned pregnancy followed by rejection by their parents. A young man's first experience of tenderness in a loving relationship may compete with the machismo assimilated from older male peers, probably including his own father. MEXFAM's videos which feature stories portraying typical conflicts between father and son on matters of sexuality and relationships, have had dramatic results with both young and older male audiences — particularly as many older men are induced to re-live the sadness they themselves experienced as young men relating to their fathers.

**Philip Meredith,** *International Planned Parenthood Federation, United Kingdom*

programme allows adolescents themselves to take a principal role in providing the information, education and services they need [41].

## MEN HAVE SEX TOO...

Despite the fact that heterosexual transmission of HIV by definition involves both men and women, some AIDS educators believe that women have been disproportionately charged with the responsibility for behaviour change within those relationships.

To control the heterosexual spread of HIV, education messages must reach both men and women. Safer sex cannot be practised by women alone. "The messages that went out to gay men in the North were being delivered to both partners. It may be that only one partner heard it — that is, only one person may have gone to a session and

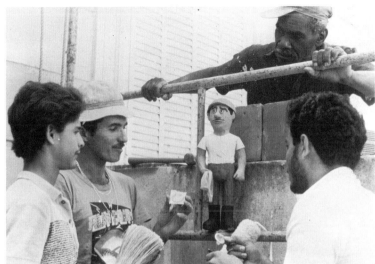

Zé Cabra-Macho does it safely. Macho Man introduces Brazilian construction workers to the practicalities of safer sex. *Brazilian Interdisciplinary AIDS Association, Rio de Janeiro, Brazil*

the other didn't — but it was a message delivered on the same understanding to both partners," says Professor Constance Wofsy, co-director of AIDS activities at San Francisco General Hospital. "With women...the messages being sent out are only going to half the partnership. Anything done to try to prevent heterosexual transmission of HIV has to be aimed at women and men....But heterosexual men by and large are not being targeted — they may be targeted coincidentally as part of a couple, the partners of sex workers say — but there's little attempt to reach men more generally through STD clinics, for example... [42]."

For women educators and counsellors the dilemma is clear. "If you're doing directive counselling as I am, what direction are we offering women?" asks Marie St Cyr, executive director of the New York-based Women's Action Resource Network. "Given that we're not educating the heterosexual male, how can we offer a woman a condom? She's not in a position where she has the power to use it...men are often not prepared to use condoms; nor are they getting the information they need to make them understand the importance of this. Because we're not targeting men and because women don't wear condoms, all studies which talk about female preference for condoms are fatally flawed... [43]"

Many men are interested in learning more about condoms but might not want to learn from their wives, say family planners involved in "male motivation" programmes who have long recognised that special attention paid to men can encourage wider and more sustained adoption of changed sexual behaviour. Men's reasons for favouring or opposing family planning often differ from those of women and

*Heterosexual men generally are not being targeted with information*

# Touting for business:
# Nigeria's STOPAIDS scheme

Since 1988, STOPAIDS has been running a pilot project to disseminate information about AIDS and other STDs to long-distance drivers using two of Nigeria's biggest inter-state motor parks. Many of the drivers spend a large part of the year in transit in Nigeria and its neighbouring countries.Some stay with different sex partners at the stop-off points en route. The project's first stage of project evaluation suggests that a proportion of those treated at the kiosk have had one or more STDs.

In each park the STOPAIDS team — made up of health officers, project officers and counsellors — operate from a small but prominently positioned "health kiosk" open six days a week. Between January and May 1990, the two kiosks were visited by about 4,000 people — mostly men.

The STOPAIDS team do not just wait for people to come to them; they go looking for customers. A key member of the team is the outreach officer, an ex-motor park ticket tout whose job it is to refer people to the kiosk. The usual job of the tout is to pick up customers for a particular company operating from the park, hence he has easy access to both "the regulars" and passengers and truckers passing through for the first time, as well as the women prostitutes who live and work on the fringes of the park.

Health officers deal with everything from bloody noses and headaches to the demonstration of effective use of condoms using a model phallus. Clients are referred to local medical centres for testing and treatment of STDs under an authorised referral procedure, sanctioned by the State Ministry of Health.

Generally treatment is free but a minimal charge is made for some routine services. To date condoms are given out free — about 15 strips of four condoms per kiosk, per day — as an incentive to encourage use. In the future they will probably be sold at subsidised and affordable rates.

"Often someone comes to the kiosk complaining of a headache but before they're finished they've admitted to thinking they've got gonorrhoea" said project director Pearl Nwashili. "We have to use whatever contact we have with the truck drivers and others to gradually introduce the issue of HIV infection and AIDS. They don't think they are at risk, so they don't ask for information. But by starting with information about other STDs — which many of them do understand because they have a history of infection — we can make them see the relevance of the risk of HIV and AIDS."

The first stage of the STOPAIDS project has concentrated on enlisting the support of the transport union leaders who are the most respected figures of authority within the parks. It is hoped that this groundwork will pay off when the pilot project is extended to cover other motor parks within Nigeria.
**Panos**

need to be discussed with other men [44]. "For example, high fertility is valued by both women and men, although not necessarily at the same time and for the same reasons," says a review of literature on sexual behaviour in sub-Saharan Africa which points to the need for more research into sexual attitudes and practice [45].

The behaviour of men as well as women is subject to complex cultural constraints. In many cultures, for example, the female kinship network of several generations can exert a powerful influence in an extended household group and is often a critical force in ensuring conformity with traditions, including those regarding family size. In

Nigeria, for example, surveys showed that while many men saw five children as the optimum family size, their wives and parents favoured eight children. Because the views of female relatives were a stronger influence on women, the larger family was often more likely [46].

Attempts have been made to reach men in factories and other work sites to teach them about safer sex and condoms [48]. The Brazilian Interdisciplinary AIDS Association has provided a prototype for AIDS prevention programmes targeted at the working man. In Rio de Janeiro, Brazil, education workers visit construction sites where hundreds of men live separated from their families for months at a time. In Mexico, education is provided within factories for the mainly male employees [49].

Some men have learned informally about AIDS prevention from women in the sex industry. In Birmingham, in the United Kingdom, one-third of the clients in one study reported learning about HIV risks and safer sex from prostitutes. Some AIDS educators are taking the message directly to the prostitutes' clients. In Cross River state, Nigeria, education sessions for prostitutes, their clients and partners are held in the hotels where the women work. The outreach to clients also relies heavily on the project's male health educator, a hotel manager. AIDS education films have also been shown in nightclubs where many part-time or occasional prostitutes meet clients. All the women are supplied with educational material for themselves and the men, and are encouraged to refer clients and partners to the project's STD clinic. Condom use by the 800 women prostitutes and 2,500 male clients in the pilot project increased by 25% in just the first three months [47].

*Behaviour in its social, economic and political context is the real challenge of the AIDS pandemic*

## NEW PRIORITIES: WOMEN SPEAK OUT

Behaviour in its social, economic and political context is the real challenge of the AIDS pandemic. "If the social, economic and cultural costs of avoiding risks are too high...women will continue to take risks with their health and reproduction," says US anthropologist Dr Dooley Worth. "Working with individual women or groups of women about sexual decision-making is not enough [50]."

It is not enough on several counts. First, because decisions within sexual relationships are taken by two people, hence HIV education must be not only for and by women, but men as well. And second, because decisions about sexual behaviour cannot be separated from the wider social and cultural influences which inform all human behaviour. HIV is not a merely medical issue, but raises the fundamental issues of equity — between the sexes and between regions of the world — which are at the heart of the development debate. Without radical change, women and particularly the most disadvantaged women in the poorest communities around the world, will remain in "triple jeopardy [51]".

Looking back over the 1980s it is clear that much of what has been said or written about AIDS has been coloured by an overwhelming, if unstated, assumption that AIDS is a disease of men. It is an assumption belied by the facts. In 1990 about a third of those infected with HIV are women, with the proportion likely to increase over the next decade. Furthermore, women are carrying most of the daily care load and managing many of the wider consequences of the pandemic in homes and hospitals around the world. Professor Constance Wofsy, co-director of AIDS activities at San Francisco General Hospital, identified women's "caring and coping" strengths as crucial in limiting the impact of AIDS. "But", she adds,"this cannot be enough. What they want is a voice — they want to be heard [52]." Without significant policy input from women, the AIDS agenda will continue to be set and run by men, largely from the North, and will fail to recognise the reality of the pandemic. Resources and research must be directed to greater understanding of how women are at risk and how they can best protect themselves.

Change is possible. Surveys and questionnaires indicate that men and women are beginning to modify or abandon behaviour which puts them at risk. Reports of reductions in the number of sexual partners and increased condom use are becoming more common. Where men traditionally have more sexual freedom, women are reportedly beginning to challenge the double standard which sanctions their partners' behaviour.

"Throughout the world there are many examples of women facing the challenges presented by HIV with strength," says US AIDS worker Kathe Karlson. "Mothers, daughters, sisters, aunts and grandmothers...sharing their experiences, acknowledging and continuing to love and care. However, their individual responses alone can never be enough for the kinds of support systems and treatments that are imperative but which have yet to be put into place [53]."

This dossier provides some examples of positive steps which women around the world are taking to protect themselves, their partners and their children from HIV infection. One common thread is that women are gaining greater control over their lives in order to be able to make informed decisions and act on them. The stronger a woman's place in society, the greater are her options for HIV prevention.

# REFERENCES

## AIDS: AN ISSUE FOR EVERY WOMAN

1. Panos interview with Sallie Perryman, special assistant to the director, AIDS Institute, New York State Department of Health, New York, June 1990.
2. Report for Panos, Amanda Heggs, Copenhagen, September 1989.
3. Interview by Catherine Watson with Miria Matembe, member of Ugandan parliament and chairperson of Action for Development (Acfode), Uganda, August 1989.
4. Report for Panos by Maru Antuñano, Puerto Rican journalist, New York, July 1990.
5. Interview with Selvi by Shyamala Nataraj, Madras, October 1989.
6. Interview with Mary by Claire Sanders in "Brief Encounters", *New Statesman & Society*, 29 June 1990, London.
7. Report for Panos by Dr Wendy Holmes, Zimbabwe, September 1989.
8. Panos interview with Marie St Cyr, executive director of the Women's Action Resource Network, New York, June 1990.
9. Information from Sheila Gilchrist, Positively Women, London, September 1990.

## CHAPTER 1: THE GLOBAL PICTURE

10. J. Chin, "Epidemiology: current and future dimensions of the HIV/AIDS pandemic in women and children", *Lancet*, 28 July 1990, Vol 336, No 8709, pp221-224.
11. "The global AIDS situation", *In Point of Fact*, June 1990, No 68, WHO.
12. D. Goldberg, "The epidemiology of HIV and AIDS in Scotland", *Abstracts of the VIth International Conference on AIDS*, San Francisco, June 1990, Th.C.722.
13. M. J. Wawer and others, "Geographic and community distribution of HIV-1 infection in rural Rakai district, Uganda", *Abstracts of VIth International Conference on AIDS*, San Francisco, June 1990, F.C.606.
14. See reference 11.
15. "WHO revises global estimates of HIV infection", *Press Release WHO/38*, 31 July 1990.
16. See reference 10.
17. Information from Dr Barry Evans, Communicable Disease Surveillance Centre, London, September 1990.
18. *HIV/AIDS Surveillance Report*, August 1990, Centers for Disease Control, Atlanta.
19. M. Gwinn and others, "Estimates of HIV seroprevalence in childbearing women and incidence of HIV infection in infants, United States", *Abstracts of VIth International Conference on AIDS*, San Francisco, June 1990, F.C.43.
20. "Face to face with drugs", *WorldAIDS*, May 1989, Panos, London , No 3.
21. See reference 18
22. J. Glaser and others, "Heterosexual human immunodeficiency virus transmission among the middle class", *Archives of Internal Medicine*, March 1989, Vol 149, No 3, pp 645-649.
23. Information from Dr George Bath, Lothian Health Board, Scotland, September 1990.
24. J. Robertson and C. Skidmore, "Heterosexually acquired HIV infection", correspondence, *British Medical Journal*, 1 April 1989, Vol 298, No 6677, p891.
25. L. Bossio and others, "Bisexuality and risk behaviour in Lima, Peru", *Abstracts of the VIth International AIDS Conference*, San Francisco, June 1990, 3005.
26. M. Carols and others, "Sexuality in women and AIDS in a Latin American country", *Abstracts of VIth International Conference on AIDS*, San Francisco, June 1990, F.C.592.
27. See reference 11.
28. E. Cortes and others, "HIV-1, HIV-2 and HTLV-1 infection in high-risk groups in Brazil", *New England Journal of Medicine*, 13 April 1989, Vol 320, No 15, pp953-958.
29. J. Valdespino, "Development of HIV/AIDS epidemic in the country ranking 4th in number of cases in the Americas", *Abstracts of VIth International Conference on AIDS*, San Francisco, June 1990, Th.C.717.
30. R. Beach and others, "HIV infection in Brazil", *New England Journal of Medicine*, 21 September 1989,

Vol 321, No 12.

31. F. Cleghorn, "Update on the epidemiology of AIDS in Trinidad", *Abstracts of VIth International Conference on AIDS*, San Francisco, June 1990, Th.C.718.

32. A. Coxon and others, "Longitudinal study of the sexual behaviour of homosexual males under the impact of AIDS", Final Report, Essex University, April 1990.

33. See reference 10.

34. See reference 15.

35. Thai Ministry of Public Health estimate quoted in J. Ungphakorn, "The impact of AIDS on women in Thailand", paper presented at "AIDS in Asia and the Pacific Conference", Canberra, August 1990.

36. See reference 10.

37. D. Smith, "Thailand: AIDS crisis looms", *Lancet*, 31 March 1990, Vol 335, pp781-782.

38. S. Apte and others, "Prevalence of anti-HIV antibodies among blood donors in Bombay", *Abstracts of the VIth International Conference on AIDS*, San Francisco, June 1990, F.C.611.

39. G. Bhave and others, "HIV sero surveillance in promiscuous females of Bombay, India", *Abstracts of the VIth International Conference on AIDS*, San Francisco, June 1990, F.C.612.

40. See reference 10.

41. "HIV-2 in perspective", Editorial, *Lancet*, 7 May 1988, Vol I, No 8593, pp1027-1028.

42. "Acquired Immunodeficiency Syndrome (AIDS): Interim proposal for a WHO staging system for HIV infection and disease", *Weekly Epidemiological Record*, 20 July 1990, No 29, pp221-224.

43. See reference 42.

44. See reference 41.

45. "No insect transmission", *WorldAIDS*, July 1990, Panos, London, No 10.

46. See reference 10.

47. A. Trebucq and others, "HIV-1 infection in males and females in Central Africa", *Lancet*, 22 July 1989, Vol 1989(ii), No 8656, pp225-226; C. Bizimungu and others, *Lancet*, 29 April 1989, Vol 1, No 8644, pp 941-943.

48. See reference 18.

49. *AIDS in New York State 1989*, State of New York Department of Health, New York, 1990.

50. "AIDS Surveillance in Europe", *Quarterly Report*, 31 March 1990, No 25, WHO Collaborating Centre, Paris.

51. "AIDS and youth", a leaflet prepared for the 1989 WHO World Health Assembly, WHO, 1989.

52. B. N'Galy and others, "HIV Prevalence in Zaire, 1984-1988", *Abstracts of IVth International Conference on AIDS*, Stockholm, June 1988, 5632.

53. A. De Schryver and A. Meheus, "Reviews/analyses, epidemiology of sexually transmitted diseases: the global picture", *Bulletin of the World Health Organization*, 1990, 68, (5), 639-654.

54. D. Burke and others, "Human immunodeficiency virus infections in teenagers: seroprevalence among applicants for US military service", *Journal of American Medical Association*, 18 April 1990, Vol 263, No 15.

55. See reference 10.

56. J. Chin, "Estimates and projections of perinatal transmission of HIV", *Abstracts of Vth International Conference on AIDS*, Montreal, June 1989, T.B.O. 18.

57. See reference 10.

58. J. Cheek and J. Chin, "HIV-infected children and AIDS-related orphans in sub-Saharan Africa", *Abstracts of VIth International Conference on AIDS*, San Francisco, June 1990, F.C. 221.

59. M. Rogers, "Update on epidemiology", *Report of The Implications of AIDS for Mothers and Children, International Conference*, Paris, November 1989.

60. See reference 18.

## CHAPTER 2: HOW ARE WOMEN AT RISK

1. N. Padian and others, "Anomalies of infectivity in heterosexual transmission of HIV", *Abstracts of the IVth International Conference on AIDS*, Stockholm, June 1988, 4062.

2. M. Al-Nozha and others, correspondence, "Female to male: an inefficient mode of transmission of human immunodeficiency virus (HIV)", *Journal of Acquired Immune Deficiency Syndrome*, February 1990, Vol 3,

No 2, pp193-194.

3. J. Wiley and others, "Heterogeneity in the probability of HIV transmission per sexual contact: the case of male-to-female transmission in penile-vaginal intercourse", *Statistics in Medicine*, 1989, Vol 8, pp 93-102.

4. See reference 2.

5. A. Johnson, "The epidemiology of HIV in the UK: sexual transmission", in *HIV and AIDS*, chapter 2, pp14-17, UK Health Department and Health Education Authority, November 1989.

6. A. Johnson and M. Laga, "Heterosexual transmission of HIV", *AIDS* 1988, 2 (suppl 1):S49-S56; A. Johnson and others, "Transmission of HIV to heterosexual partners of infected men and women", *AIDS* 1989, pp3367-3372.

7. W. Cameron and others, "Female to male transmission of human immunodeficiency virus type 1:riskfactors for seroconversion in men", *New England Journal of Medicine*, August 17 1989, Vol 321, No7, p403.

8. See reference 5.

9. C. Garcia Moreno, "Women and AIDS", Oxfam (Health Unit) Information Sheet, Oxford, February 1989.

10. F. Chiodo and others, "Risk factors in heterosexual transmission of HIV", *Abstracts of the VIth International Conference on AIDS*, San Francisco, June 1990, Th.C.583.

11. N. Padian and others, "Male to female transmission of human immunodeficiency virus", *Journal of the American Medical Association*, 1987, 258:788-91.

12. Michael Marmor and others, "Possible female to female transmission of HIV", *Annals of Internal Medicine*, 1986, Vol 105, p969.

13. P. Spitzer and N. Weiner, "Transmission of HIV infection from a woman to a man by oral sex," *New England Journal of Medicine*, 26 January 1989, Vol 320, No 4, p251.

14. Marea Murray, "Dental dams debunked", *Sexual Health Report*, Spring 1988, Vol 9, quoted in report for Panos by Heather Downs, Terrence Higgins Trust Women's Group, London, June 1990.

15. Panos interview with Dr Francis Plummer, University of Manitoba, Canada, June 1988.

16. D.W. Cameron and others, "Incidence and risk factors for female to male transmission of HIV", *Abstracts of the IVth International Conference on AIDS*, Stockholm, June 1988, 4061.

17. M. Laga, "Non ulcerative sexually transmitted diseases (STD) as risk factors for HIV infection", *Abstracts of the VIth International Conference on AIDS*, Th.C.97; J. Ombette and others, "Presence of HIV among men and women with H. ducreyi and Neisseria gonorrhoeae infection in Nairobi, Kenya", *Abstracts of the VIth International Conference on AIDS*, San Francisco, June 1990, Th.C.572.

18. A. De Schryver and A. Meheus, "Reviews/analyses, epidemiology of sexually transmitted diseases: the global picture", *Bulletin of the World Health Organization*, 1990, 68, (5): 639-654.

19. "Let's unite against AIDS", Report of the First Workshop of the Society for Women and AIDS in Africa (SWAA), Harare, May 1989.

20. See reference 7.

21. J. Simonson and others, "HIV infection among lower socioeconomic strata prostitutes in Nairobi", *AIDS*, 1990, Vol 4, No 2, pp139-144.

22. Contraceptive methods and human immunodeficiency virus (HIV), WHO/SPA/INF/87.9, WHO, Geneva, 1987.

23. Report for Panos by Dr Hanne Friesen, Save The Children Fund, Uganda, September 1989.

24. Information from Dr James Chin, WHO, GPA, September 1990.

25. Information from Pat Corcoran, WHO, September 1990.

26. Report for Panos by Shyamala Nataraj, Madras, August 1990.

27. Report for Panos by Heather Downs, Terrence Higgins Trust Women's Group, London, August 1990.

28. D. Worth, "Sexual decision-making and AIDS: why condom promotion among vulnerable women is likely to fail," *Studies in Family Planning*, Nov/Dec 1989, Vol 20, No 6, pp297-307.

29. H. Ward and others, "HIV risk behaviour and STD incidence in London prostitutes", *Abstracts of the VIth International Conference on AIDS*, San Francisco, June 1990, F.C.738.

30. See reference 28.

31. Claire Sanders, "Dangerous Liaisons", *New Statesman & Society*, 6 July 1990, London.

32. S. Saltzman and others, "Factors associated with recurrence of unsafe sex practices in a cohort of gay men previously engaging in 'safer sex'", *Abstracts of the Vth International Conference on AIDS*, Montreal, June 1989, T.D.P.31.

# CHAPTER 3: A QUESTION OF CHOICE

1. Dr Eustace Muhondwa, Dept of Behavioural Sciences, University of Tanzania, plenary presentation, VIth International Conference on AIDS, San Francisco, June 1990.
2. Dr A. Nasidi, Federal Vaccine Production Laboratory, Lagos, comments following "HIV infection in polygamous families in Nigeria", paper presented at the Second SWAA Workshop, Lagos, May 1990.
3. N. Freudenberg, "Social and political obstacles to AIDS education", *SIECUS Report*, August/September 1989, Vol 17, No 6, Sex Information and Education Council of the US, New York.
4. R. Selverstone, "Where are we now in the sexual revolution?", *SIECUS Report*, March/April 1989, Vol 17, No 2, Sex Information and Education Council of the US, New York.
5. Cited in D. Burke and others, "Human immunodeficiency virus infections in teenagers: seroprevalence among applicants for US military service", *Journal of the American Medical Association*, 18 April 1990, Vol 263, No 15, pp2074-2077.
6. Elise Jones and others, *Teenage Pregnancy in Industrialized Countries*, Yale University Press, New Haven, 1986.
7. D. Worth, "Sexual decision-making and AIDS: why condom promotion among vulnerable women is likely to fail", *Studies in Family Planning*, Nov/Dec 1989, Vol 20, No 6, pp297-307.
8. M. Jingu, "High condom utilization and low seroconversion rates successfully sustained in 175 married couples in Zaire with discordant serology; observations after two years of follow-up", *Abstracts of the VIth International Conference on AIDS*, San Francisco, June 1990, S.C.695.
9. S. Cochran and V. Mays, "Sex, lies and HIV", correspondence, *New England Journal of Medicine*, 15 March 1990, Vol 322, No 11, p774.
10. Chantawipa Apisook & Elain McDonnell, "Thailand: the 'foreign' disease", *The Third Epidemic*, Panos, London, 1990, p204.
11. Hilary Kinnell, "Prostitutes, their clients and risks of HIV infection in Birmingham", Central Birmingham Health Authority, UK, revised edition August 1989.
12. Report for Panos by Dr Geoff Foster, president, Family AIDS Counselling Trust (FACT), Zimbabwe, May 1990.
13. Dr Jose Marti Nunez, gynaecologist, Head of Interagency Coordinating Council for AIDS in Puerto Rico (COMINSIDA), quoted in a Report for Panos by Vincent Gil, Professor of Human Sexuality and Anthropology, Southern California College, USA, November 1989.
14. Michael Marmor and others, "Possible female to female transmission of HIV", *Annals of Internal Medicine*, 1989, Vol 105: 969; O.T. Monzon & J.M.B. Capellan, "Female to female transmission of HIV", *Lancet*, 4 July 1987, Vol II, No 8549, pp40-42.
15. Johannes F. Linn, *Cities in the developing world*, Oxford University Press, Oxford, 1983, pxiii.
16. Jorge Hardoy and David Satterthwaite, *Squatter Citizen*, Earthscan, London, 1989, p5.
17. "Let's unite against AIDS", Report of the First Workshop of the Society for Women and AIDS in Africa (SWAA), Harare, May 1989.
18. Edda Ivan-Smith and others, *Women in Sub-Saharan Africa*, London, Minority Rights Group, 1988, p5.
19. J. Ungphakorn, "The impact of AIDS on women in Thailand", paper presented to the AIDS in Asia and the Pacific Conference, Canberra, August 1990.
20. "Coping with the impact of AIDS on women in Africa", Report of the Second Workshop of the Society for Women and AIDS in Africa (SWAA), Lagos, May 1990.
21. G. Williams (ed), *Fear to Hope: AIDS Care and Prevention at Chikankata Hosptial, Zambia*, Strategies for Hope, No 1, ActionAid, London, February 1990, p21.
22. Information from Dr Mukesh Kapila, Health Education Authority, London, September 1990.
23. H. I. Goldberg and others, "Knowledge about condoms and their use in less developed countries during a period of rising AIDS prevalence", *Bulletin of the World Health Organization* 1989, 67:1, pp85-91.
24. Report for Panos by Marge Berer, Women's Global Network on Reproductive Rights, Amsterdam, June 1990.
25. *CDC AIDS Weekly*, 17 July 1989, CDC AIDS WEEKLY, Birmingham, Alabama, US.
26. Panos interview with Dr Edwige Bienvenu-Ba, University of Dakar, Senegal, May 1990.
27. *AIDSWatch* 1989, No 6, 2nd quarter, International Planned Parenthood Federation, London.
28. "Churches in Africa: joining in the battle against AIDS", September 1989, Document No 14, Ecumenical

Documentation and Information Centre for Eastern and Southern Africa, Zimbabwe.

29. H. I. Goldberg and others, "Knowledge about condoms and their use in less developed countries during a period of rising AIDS prevalence", *Bulletin of the World Health Organization*, 1989, 67:1, pp85-91 quoted in Report for Panos by Marge Berer, Women's Global Network on Reproductive Rights, Amsterdam, June 1990.

30. Report for Panos by Jane Galvao, Executive Secretary, Religious Support Against AIDS (ARCA), Brazil, August 1990.

31. M. Leeper, "Update of WPC-333 female condom clinical results", *Abstracts of the VIth International Conference on AIDS*, San Francisco, June 1990, S.C.758.

32. Information from Mary Ann Leeper, director of Product Development, Wisconsin Pharmacal, US, August 1990.

33. C. Bradbeer, "Women and HIV", *British Medical Journal*, 11 February 1989, Vol 298: 342-343.

34. M. Rekart and others, "Nonoxynol 9: its adverse effects", *Abstracts of the VIth International Conference on AIDS*, San Francisco, June 1990, S.C.36.

35. J. Kreiss and others, "Efficacy of Nonoxynol-9 in preventing HIV transmission", *Abstracts from the Vth International Conference on AIDS*, Montreal, June 1989, M.A.O.36.

36. Ceri Hutton, "Bed etiquette", *New Statesman & Society*, 6 July 1990, London.

37. Gloria Mock, quoted in Report for Panos by Vincent Gill, Professor of Human Sexuality and Anthropology, Southern California College, California, November 1989.

38. See reference 30.

39. Claire Sanders, "Dangerous Liaisons", *New Statesman & Society*, 6 July 1990, London.

40. See reference 17

41. Panos interview with Carmen Chavez, Latino AIDS Project, Instituto Familiar de la Raza, San Francisco, November 1988.

42. See reference 7.

43. *The Observer*, London, 19 August 1990.

44. S-Y. Yoon, "Asian women and AIDS: research issues", *Abstracts of the Vth International Conference on AIDS*, Montreal, June 1989, D.695.

45. Comment from the floor, Second SWAA Workshop, Lagos, May 1990.

46. M. Weiner and others, "Change in AIDS knowledge, perceptions and risk practices for female partners of IV drug users after educational interventions: initial findings", *Abstracts of the VIth International Conference on AIDS*, San Francisco, June 1990, S.C.751.

47. Panos interview with Sallie Perryman, special assistant to the director, AIDS Institute, New York State Department of Health, New York, June 1990.

48. Panos interview with Professor Constance Wofsy, co-director of AIDS Activities at San Francisco General Hospital, San Francisco, June 1990.

49. K. Siegel, "Public education to prevent the spread of HIV infection", *New York State Journal of Medicine*, December 1988: 642-646.

50. See reference 24.

51. See reference 7.

52. Panos interview with Marie St Cyr, executive director, Women's Action Resource Network (WARN), New York, June 1990.

53. R. Eversley, "AIDS intervention in psychotherapeutic practice with high risk minority women", paper presented at IVth International Conference on AIDS, Stockholm, June 1988.

54. *New York Times*, New York, 27 August 1987.

55. See reference 7.

56. See reference 19.

57. Vern Bullough and Bonnie Bullough, *Women and Prostitution: A social history*, New York, Prometheus Books, 1989, p296.

58. See reference 19; and *Nation*, Bangkok, 13 September 1987.

59. Dr John Chikwem, at the Second SWAA Workshop, Lagos, May 1990.

60. Priscilla Alexander, "Prostitutes and AIDS: public policy considerations, testimony before the president's commission on AIDS", COYOTE, National Task Force on Prostitution, US, 24 March 1988.

61. "Don't Die of Ignorance — I nearly died of embarrassment: Condoms in Context", paper presented by the Women, Risk and AIDS Project at the Fourth Social Aspects of AIDS Conference, London, April 1990.

## CHAPTER 4: HIV INFECTION, REPRODUCTION AND MOTHERHOOOD

1. Report for Panos by Amanda Heggs, Copenhagen, September 1989.

2. Panos interview with Professor Constance Wofsy, co-director AIDS Activities, San Francisco General Hospital, San Francisco, June 1990.

3. A. Willoughby, "Clinical science and trials", rapporteur session, *Abstracts of VIth International Conference on AIDS*, San Francisco, June 1990.

4. W. Friedman and others, "Increased frequency of cervical dysplasia/neoplasia in HIV-infected women is related to the extent of immunosuppression", *Abstracts of VIth International Conference on AIDS*, San Francisco, June 1990, S.B.519; S. Vermund and others, "Risk of human papillomavirus (HPV) and cervical squamous intraepithelial lesions (SIL) highest among women with advanced HIV disease", *Abstracts of VIth International Conference on AIDS*, San Francisco, June 1990, S.B.517.

5. C. Marta and others, "Need for gynaecologic protocols in AIDS primary care clinics", *Abstracts of Vth International Conference on AIDS*, Montreal, June 1989, M.B.P.276.

6. Information from Dr Peter Selwyn, Montefiore Medical Centre, New York, August 1990.

7. P. Wambugu and others, "Clinical manifestations of HIV-1 infection among women working as prostitutes in Nairobi", *Abstracts of the VIth International Conference on AIDS*, San Francisco, June 1990, Th.C.543.

8. See reference 3.

9. E. Mbidde and others, "The epidemiology and clinical features of Kaposi's sarcoma (KS) in African women with HIV infection", *Abstracts of VIth International Conference on AIDS*, San Francisco, June 1990, S.B.508.

10. Report for Panos by Kathe Karlson, Upper Manhattan Task Force on AIDS, New York, September 1990.

11. See reference 5.

12. R. Rothenberg and others, *New England Journal of Medicine*, 19 November 1987, Vol 317, No 21, pp1297-1301.

13. See reference 6.

14. Panos Interview with Katie Bias, Women's Outreach Network of the National Haemophilia Foundation, US, June 1990.

15. J. Maurice, "Women and tropical diseases", *Tropical Disease Research (TDR) News*, June 1989, No 28, WHO.

16. A. Berrebi and others, "Influence of gestation on HIV infection," *Abstracts of VIth International Conference on AIDS*, San Francisco, June 1990, Th.C. 651; K. Bledscoe and others, "Effect of pregnancy on progression of HIV infection", *Abstracts of VIth International Conference on AIDS*, San Francisco, June 1990, Th.C.652.

17. J. Bury, "Counselling women with HIV infection about pregnancy, heterosexual transmission and contraception", *The British Journal of Family Planning*, January 1989, Vol 14, No 4, pp116-22.

18. R. Weber, "Cessation of intravenous drug use reduces progression of HIV infection in HIV-positive drug users", *Abstracts of VIth International Conference on AIDS*, San Francisco, June 1990, Th.C.36.

19. L. Hauer, "Pregnancy and HIV infection. Focus: a guide to AIDS research and counselling", University of California at San Francisco, AIDS Health Project, San Francisco, October 1989, pp1-2.

20. Mark Crawford (ed), "Briefings: treatment lacking for pregnant addicts," *Science*, 19 January 1990, Vol 247, pp257-372.

21. S. Blanche and others, "A prospective study of infants born to women seropositive for HIV1", *New England Journal of Medicine*, 22 June 1989, Vol 320, No 25, pp1643-8.

22. A. Poulsen and others, "No evidence of vertical transmission of HIV-2 in Bissau", *Abstracts of the Vth International Conference on AIDS*, Montreal, June 1989, T.G.P.31.

23. Presentation by Dr Richard Tedder to the UK NGO Consortium on AIDS and the Third World, London, July 1989.

24. See reference 21

25. P.Tovo and M. de Martino, "Epidemiology and natural history of HIV infection in children, Results from

the Italian multicentre study on 1316 subjects", *Abstracts of VIth International Conference on AIDS*, San Francisco, June 1990, Th.C.660.

26. P. Lepage, "Natural history of HIV-1 infection in African children, A prospective cohort study in Rwanda", *Abstracts of VIth International Conference on AIDS*, San Francisco, June 1990, Th.C. 659.

27. Information from Dr M.L. Newell, Institute of Child Health, London, September 1990.

28. T. Manzila and others, "Perinatally acquired HIV infection (P1): absence of an additional risk due to breast feeding in a cohort of 108 infants born to HIV(+) mothers", *Abstracts of The Implications of AIDS for Mothers and Children International Conference*, Paris, November 1989, B2.

29. N. Halsey and others, "Maternal-infant HIV-1 transmission (MIT) in breastfed Haitian infants", *Abstracts of VIth International Conference on AIDS*, San Francisco, June 1990, Th.C.609.

30. Statement from the consultation on breast-feeding/breast milk and human immunodeficiency virus (HIV), WHO/SPA/INF/87.8, WHO, Geneva, 23-25 June 1987.

31. P. M'pélé and others, "Knowledge and attitudes: mother to child transmission of HIV1 and prenatal screening in Brazzaville (Congo)", *Abstracts of the First International Symposium on Education and Information about AIDS*, 16-20 October 1988, Ixtapa, Mexico, RT3-41.

32. H. Minkoff and others, "Routinely offered prenatal HIV testing", correspondence, *New England Journal of Medicine*, 13 October 1988, Vol 319, No 15, p1018.

33. K. Krasinski and others, "Failure of voluntary testing for human immunodeficiency virus to identify infected parturient women in a high-risk population", *New England Journal of Medicine*, 21 January 1988, Vol 318, No 3, p185.

34. H. Hull and others, "Comparison of HIV-antibody prevalence in patients consenting to and declining HIV antibody testing in an STD clinic", *Journal of the American Medical Association*, 19 August 1988, Vol 260, No 7, pp935-938.

35. See reference 19.

36. See reference 14.

37. "My Story: Three Scenarios", *AIDS: An Issue for Every Woman*, Report of the Women and AIDS Support Network Conference, Harare, Zimbabwe, 1990".

38. U. Jakobs, "Psychological support for HIV-infected female patients in coping with critical life-events in gynaecology and obstetrics", *Abstracts of VIth International Conference on AIDS*, San Francisco, June 1990, S.D.819.

39. K. Franke, "Discrimination against HIV-positive women by abortion clinics in New York City", *Abstracts of Vth International Conference on AIDS*, Montreal, June 1989, T.E.P. 52.

40. L. Mofenson and others, "Prenatal screening policies for HIV antibodies at major obstetric clinical centers in the United States", *Abstracts of VIth International Conference on AIDS*, San Francisco, June 1990, S.C. 665; F. Johnstone and others, "Women's knowledge of their HIV antibody state: its effect on their decision whether to continue the pregnancy", *British Medical Journal*, 6 January 1990, Vol 300, No 6716, pp23-24.

41. J. Arras, "Should HIV positive women have children? An ethical perspective", *Abstracts of the Vth International Conference on AIDS*, Montreal, June 1989, T.F.O.19.

42. See reference 19.

43. J. Mitchell, "Women, AIDS and public policy", *AIDS and Public Policy Journal*, 1988, Vol 3, No 2.

44. M. Foreman and others, "HIV-positive women infected though intravenous drug use in Ireland and their future plans for themselves and their children", *Abstracts of the VIth International Conference on AIDS*, San Francisco, June 1990, Th.D.799.

45. N. Badi and others, "Poor sustainability of birth control utilization and consequent high fertility rates in a cohort of 249 HIV(+) Zairian women aware of their serostatus and followed for 30 months post-partum", *Abstracts of the VIth International Conference on AIDS*, San Francisco, June 1990, Th.D.121.

46. Judith Bury, "Counselling women with HIV infection about pregnancy, heterosexual transmission and contraception", *The British Journal of Family Planning*, January 1989, Vol 14, No 4, pp116-22.

47. W. Crombleholme, "Perinatal HIV transmission despite maternal/infant AZT therapy", *Abstracts of the VIth International Conference on AIDS*, San Francisco, June 1990, Th.C.605.

48. P. Selwyn and others, "Knowledge of HIV antibody status and decisions to continue or terminate pregnancy among intravenous drug users", *Journal of the American Medical Association*, June 1989, Vol 261, No 24, pp3567-71; and information from Dr Ann Marie Kimball, Pan American Health Organization,

Washington, June 1990.

49. G. Williams (ed), *From Fear to Hope: AIDS Care and Prevention at Chikankata Hospital, Zambia*, Strategies for Hope No 1, ActionAid, London, February 1990.

50. J. Mitchell, "Strategies of prevention of perinatal transmission", plenary presentation, VIth International Conference on AIDS, San Francisco, June 1990.

51. See reference 17.

52. Information from Dr Gabe Bialy, Head of Contraceptive Development Branch, National Institutes of Health, US, August 1990.

53. P. Selwyn and others, "Knowledge of HIV antibody status and decisions to continue or terminate pregnancy among intravenous drug users", *Journal of the American Medical Association*, June 1989, Vol 261, No 24.

54. See reference 19.

55. Report for Panos by Priscilla Alexander, former co-director COYOTE, the National Task Force on Prostitution, California, June 1990.

56. M. Amanyire Byangire, "Mobilising Women for AIDS Prevention and Control", paper presented at the second SWAA workshop, Lagos, May 1990.

57. N. Lusakulira and others, "The social impact of HIV infection in the Zaire population", *Abstracts of AIDS and Associated Cancers in Africa*, October 1988, Arusha, Tanzania, P.S.6.7.

58. Editorial, "Human immunodeficiency virus in women", *Journal of the American Medical Association*, 17 April 1987, Vol 257, No 15, pp2074-2076.

59. N. Kaleeba, "A family commitment", *AIDS Action*, June 1989, Appropriate Health Resources & Technologies Action Group, (AHRTAG), London, No 7.

60. Information from HIV-positive woman, anonymous, August 1990.

61. Report for Panos by Amanda Heggs, Copenhagen, September 1989.

62. Panos interview with Sheila Gilchrist and Caroline Guinness, Positively Women, London, June 1989.

63. "AIDS: An Issue for Every woman", report of the Women and AIDS Support Network Conference, Harare, Zimbabwe, November 1989.

64. "My husband gave me HIV", *The Independent*, London, 29 November 1988.

65. Marie St Cyr, "Parallel track: Issues of access and availabilty for women and people of colour", paper presented at the VIth International Conference on AIDS, San Francisco, June 1990.

66. Jayne Garrison , "Hassled out of drug trials, she treats herself", *San Francisco Examiner*, San Francisco, 23 June 1990.

67. J. Mitchell, "Strategies for prevention of perinatal transmission", plenary presentation, VIth International Conference on AIDS, San Francisco, June 1990.

68. See reference 3.

69. See reference 19.

70. See reference 2.

71. See reference 65

72. E. Katabira, "Clinical trials in the developing world", plenary presentation, VIth International Conference on AIDS, San Francisco, June 1990.

73. Dr Eustace Muhondwa, "International scientific collaboration research — by whom and for what?", plenary presentation, VIth International Conference on AIDS, San Francisco, June 1990.

## CHAPTER 5: HIV DISEASE IN INFANTS

1. I. Kuznetsova, "Transmission of HIV-infection from an infected infant to his mother by breast feeding", *Abstracts of VIth International Conference on AIDS*, San Francisco, June 1990, Th.C.48.

2. Nicolae Beldescu, "Nosocomial transmission of HIV in Romania", Ministry of Health, Romania, paper presented at the VIth International Conference on AIDS, San Francisco, June 1990.

3. C. Almedal, "Romania's hidden epidemic", *WorldAIDS*, March 1990, Panos, London, No 8.

4. M. Radlett, "AIDS and the Third World: Guarding Against Deadly Blood", *Panoscope*, May 1989, Panos, London, No 12.

5. F. Davachi and others, "Effects of an educational campaign to reduce blood transfusions in children in Kinshasa, Zaire", *Abstracts of the Vth International Conference on AIDS*, Montreal, June 1989, E666.

6. Shilalukey Ngoma, Consultant Paediatrician/Neonatologist, University Teaching Hospital Lusaka, at the Second SWAA Workshop, Lagos, May 1990.

7. J. Chin, "Epidemiology: current and future dimensions of the HIV/AIDS pandemic in women and children", *Lancet*, 28 July 1990, Vol 336, No 8709, pp221-224.

8. I. Auger, "Incubation periods for paediatric AIDS patients", *Nature*, 8 December 1988, Vol 336, pp575-7.

9. D. Costagliola, "Incubation time for Aids among homosexual and pediatric cases", *Abstracts of the VIth International Conference on AIDS*, San Francisco, June 1990, TH.C.661.

10. Information from Dr Andrea Kovacs, Los Angeles County and University of South California Medical Centre, Los Angeles, September 1990.

11. See reference 9.

12. See reference 10.

13. H. Burger and others, "Long HIV-1 incubation periods and dynamics of transmission within a family", *Lancet*, 21 July 1990, Vol 336, No 8708, pp134-136.

14. K. Shah and others, "Changing face of perinatal infection: initial presentation at or after 5 years of age", *Abstracts of VIth International Conference on AIDS*, San Francisco, June 1990, F.B.471.

15. Sally Squires, "Treatment lag for children with AIDS", *International Herald Tribune*, March 2 1989, Paris.

16. M. Grodin and W. Mariner, "Newborns as research subjects in AIDS drug trials under ambiguous federal regulations", *Abstracts of VIth International Conference on AIDS*, San Francisco, June 1990, Th.D.807.

17. *Wall Street Journal*, 20 April 1988, New York.

## CHAPTER 6: WHO CARES, WHO PAYS?

1. Helena Pizurki and others, *Women as Providers of Health Care*, WHO, Geneva, 1987, p17.

2. Ruth Leger Sivard, *Women... A World Survey*, World Priorities, Washington, 1985, p11.

3. Report for Panos by Dr Marie Thérèse Feuerstein, freelance consultant on health issues, London, May 1990.

4. Panos interview with Noerine Kaleeba, director, The AIDS Support Organisation of Uganda (TASO), Lagos, May 1990.

5. Nina Glick Schiller and others, "The role of kin in care giving for persons with AIDS in New Jersey", *Abstracts of the VIth International Conference on AIDS*, San Francisco, June 1990, TH.D.822.

6. Report for Panos by Jane Galvao, executive secretary, Religious Support Against AIDS, Brazil, August 1990.

7. A. Dunn and S. Hunter, "Uganda, AIDS and families", *Is AIDS a development issue?*, December 1989, UK NGO AIDS Consortium for the Third World, London.

8. E. Ngugi, "Caring: the cost to a community", *WorldAIDS*, March 1990, Panos, London, No 8.

9. See reference 4.

10. T. Barnett and others, *Development Forum*, November/December 1988, No 15.

11. S. Gillespie, "Potential impact of AIDS on farming systems: a case study from Rwanda", *Land Use Policy*, 1989, Vol 6, No 4, pp301-312.

12. T. Barnett and Piers Blaikie, "Communities cope by adapting agriculture", *WorldAIDS*, March 1990, Panos, London, No 8.

13. S. Hassig and others, "The economic impact of HIV infection in adult admissions to internal medicine at Mama Yemo Hospital", *Abstracts of the Vth International Conference on AIDS*, Montreal, June 1989, T.H.09.

14. "Fighting on home ground", *WorldAIDS*, July 1989, Panos, London, No 4.

15. Jeff Montforti, "Advocating for children with HIV and their Families", speech given at VIth International Conference on AIDS, San Francisco, June 1990.

16. J. Seibert, "Paediatric AIDS: Psychosocial Issues", paper presented at the Perspectives on Paediatric AIDS Symposium at the 96th Annual Convention of the American Psychological Association, Atlanta, Georgia, August 1988.

17. W. Goeren and others, "Case management of families with HIV Infection", *Abstracts of the VIth International Conference on AIDS*, San Francisco, June 1990, S.D.803.

18. Panos interview with Sallie Perryman, special assistant to the director, AIDS Institute, New York ate Department of Health, New York, June 1990.

19. Brigid Caffrey and others, "An effective approach to providing comprehensive treatment for the

HIV-infected child: 'one stop shopping'", *Abstracts of the VIth International Conference on AIDS*, San Francisco, June 1990, 4029.

20. G. Feleke, "The role of a visiting physician in an AIDS care programme", *Abstracts of the VIth International Conference on AIDS*, San Francisco, June 1990, 4021.

21. Simon Mansfield, "The role of a hospital based home care team in the care of people with HIV disease", *Abstracts of the VIth International Conference on AIDS*, San Francisco, June 1990, S.D. 817.

22. Panos interview with Katie Bias, Women's Outreach Network of the National Haemophilia Foundation, USA, June 1990.

23. "Interactive training series for caregivers of HIV infected children", *Abstracts of the VIth International Conference on AIDS*, San Francisco, June 1990, Th.D.816.

24. Adell Harris, "Treating the uninfected sibling", *Abstracts of the VIth International Conference on AIDS*, San Francisco, June 1990, Th.D.123.

25. Panos interview with John O'Rourke, director, Parents' Paediatric AIDS Coalition , San Francisco, June 1990.

26. Panos interview with Marilyn Robinson, Center for Attitudinal Healing, California, USA, June 1988.

27. See reference 18.

28. Susan Garceau, "Survey results on how tolerant, caring and compassionate Canadians are towards those most affected by AIDS", *Abstracts of the VIth International Conference on AIDS*, San Francisco, June 1990, Th.D.844.

29. Sharon McDonald, "Tender Loving Care", *The Advocate*, 3 January 1989 reporting on Mothers of AIDS Patients (MAP), a Los Angeles area group.

30. See reference 4.

31. J. Chin, "Epidemiology: current and future dimensions of the HIV/AIDS pandemic in women and children", *Lancet*, 28 July 1990, Vol 336, No 8709, pp221-224.

32. Jane Perlez, "In Uganda district, AIDS orphans struggle to survive", *New York Times*, 10 June 1990, New York.

33. Charles Mmbaga, "AIDS Increases Orphans", *The Times of Swaziland*, 4 April 1990, Mbabne, Swaziland.

34. Bruce Lambert, "Huge by-product of AIDS is emerging: a generation of thousands of orphans", *International Herald Tribune*, 1 August 1989, Paris.

35. Phyllis Gurdin, "Adoption as a life-plan for HIV positive children", *Abstracts of the VIth International Conference on AIDS*, San Francisco, June 1990, Th.D.128.

36. Information from Sister Marty, Starcross Lay Catholic Community, Annapolis, California, September 1988.

37. Jonathan Mann, "Global AIDS: revolution, paradigm and solidarity", speech at the *VIth International Conference on AIDS*, San Francisco, June 1990.

38. *UNICEF: The state of the world's children 1989*, Oxford University Press, Oxford, 1989.

39. "Zidovudine for symptomless HIV infection", Editorial, *Lancet*, 7 April 1990, Vol 335, No 8693, pp821-822.

40. Henry Aaron and William Schwartz, "Rationing health care: the choice before us", *Science*, 26 January 1990, Vol 247, pp418- 422.

41. Dan Greenberg, "Washington perspective, who pays for health care?", *Lancet*, 3 February 1990, Vol 335, No 8684, pp280-281.

42. N. Hunter-Young, "Patterns of discharge delay and resulting financial impact for AIDS related admissions", *Abstracts of the VIth International Conference on AIDS*, San Francisco, June 1990, F.D.809.

43. R. Tapia-Conyer and others, "Estimation of AIDS treatment cost through a prospective study", *Abstracts of the VIth International Conference on AIDS*, San Francisco, June 1990, F.D.804.

44. Elizabeth Hintz and others, "Care and treatment of pediatric AIDS patients in children's hospitals", *Abstracts of the VIth International Conference on AIDS*, San Francisco, June 1990, F.D.822.

45. *AIDS Policy and the Law*, 19 October 1988, Vol 3, No 19.

46. *AIDS & Children: A family disease*, Panos, London, November 1989, p5.

47. See reference 3.

48. Fernanda Ramos, at the Second SWAA Workshop, Lagos, May 1990.

49. Susan Rifkin and Gill Walt, "Why health improves: defining the issues concerning 'comprehensive primary

health care' and 'selective primary health care'", *Social Science and Medicine*, 1986, Vol 23, No 6.

50. Powell-Cope, "Family caregivers of PWAs: experiences with health care providers", *Abstracts of the VIth International Conference on AIDS*, San Francisco, June 1990, Th.D.819.

51. Presentation by Mildred Pearson at the International Ecumencial Consultation on the Churches and AIDS, convened by the Panos Institute, Washington, March 1990.

## CHAPTER 7: AIDS PREVENTION AND THE STATUS OF WOMEN

1. "Women, mothers, children and global AIDS", special issue, *Global AIDS Factfile, GPA Digest*, December 1989, WHO.

2. M. Becket and others,"Behavioural change to reduce risk", *American Journal of Public Health*, April 1988, Vol 78, No 4, p394.

3. Ruth Leger Sivard, *Women ...A World Survey*, World Priorities, Washington, 1985, p16 .

4. "Can community carers cope?", *WorldAIDS*, July 1989, Panos, London, No 4.

5. See Reference 1.

6. M. Ladjali and P. Huston, "Listen to women first", *People*, 1990, Vol 17, No 1.

7. C. O'Gara and R. Landis, "Designing AIDS-control interventions for women: give us the tools and we will do the job", *Abstracts of the First International Symposium on Education and Information about AIDS*, Ixtapa, Mexico, October 1988.

8. Report for Panos by Marge Berer, Women's Global Network on Reproductive Rights, Amsterdam, June 1990.

9. R. Schwartz, "Developing innovative structures to reach women at high risk for HIV infection", *Abstracts of the First International Symposium on education and information about AIDS*, Ixtapa, Mexico, October 1988, pp3-97.

10. Panos interview with Sheila Gilchrist and Caroline Guinness, Positively Women, UK, June 1989.

11. Interview with Katie Bias, Women's Outreach Network of the National Haemophilia Foundation, US, June 1990.

12. Interview with Sallie Perryman, special assistant to the director, AIDS Institute, New York State Department of Health, New York, June 1990.

13. D. Taylor, "The evolution of dignity: role of Cook county hospital (CCH) support group for HIV-infected women", *Abstracts of the VIth International Conference on AIDS*, San Francisco, June 1990, Th.D.798.

14. Report for Panos by Jacalyn Lee, Hunter College of Cuny, School of Health Sciences, New York, September 1989.

15. H. Hughes, "Raising awareness of AIDS amongst Haiti's poor", *Oxfam News*, Summer 1990, Oxford.

16. Josephina Vidal, "Laundromat Lessons", *WorldAIDS*, March 1989, Panos, London, No 2.

17. "Coping with the impact of AIDS on Women in Africa", Report of the Second Workshop of the Society for Women and AIDS in Africa (SWAA), Lagos, May 1990.

18. Report for Panos by Jane Galvao, executive secretary, Religious Support Against AIDS, Rio de Janeiro, Brazil, August 1990.

19. *Child Survival Action News*, Nov-Dec 1987, no 8.

20. See reference 6.

21. Philip Meredith, *Male involvement in planned parenthood: global review and strategies for programme development*, IPPF, London, 1989.

22. "Promoting safer sex: the prevention of AIDS and other STDs", International Workshop Report, Netherlands STD Foundation, April 30-May 3 1989, p3-4.

23. Panos interview with Cheryl Overs, Victoria Prostitutes' Collective, Victoria, Australia, June 1990.

24. Report for Panos by Priscilla Alexander, former co-director, COYOTE, the National Task force on Prostitution, California, June 1990.

25. C. Overs, "AIDS prevention in the legalized sex industry", *Abstracts of the Vth International Conference on AIDS*, Montreal, June 1989, Th.D.P.91.

26. J. Chikwem and others, "Human immunodeficiency virus type 1 (HIV-1) infection among female prostitutes in Borno State of Nigeria — one year follow-up", *East African Medical Journal*, Vol 66, 742-746, 1989.

27. Report for Panos by Colleen Lowe Morna, Ghana, April 1989.

28. See reference 27.

29. Diane Smith, "Green cards for Thai sex workers", *WorldAIDS*, July 1990, Panos, London, No 10.

30. "Sexually transmitted diseases and prostitution", press release WHO/42, 31 October 1988.

31. C. R. Manaloto and others, "Sexual behaviour of Filipino female prostitutes after diagnosis of HIV infection", paper presented at 2nd International Congress on AIDS in Asia, Bangkok, Thailand, January 1989.

32. See reference 29.

33. See reference 10.

34. Report for Panos by Vincent Gil, Professor of Human Sexuality and Anthropology, Southern California College, California, November 1989.

35. Lynn Peterson, "The issue — and controversy — surrounding adolescent sexuality and abstinence", *SIECUS Report*, Sept/Oct 1988, Vol 17, No 1, Sex Information and Education Council of the US, New York.

36. Sexuality education study, highlights from relevant surveys 1988-1990, *SIECUS Report*, Dec 1989/Jan 1990, Vol 18, No 2, Sex Information and Education Council of the US, New York.

37. D. Haffner, "AIDS and Adolescents: the time for prevention is now", The Center for Population Options, Washington, November 1987.

38. Panos interview with Noerine Kaleeba, director, The AIDS Support Organisation of Uganda (TASO), Lagos, May 1990.

39. Mary Amanyire Byangire, "Mobilising Women for AIDS Prevention and Control", comment following paper presented at the Second SWAA Workshop, Lagos, May 1990.

40. Report for Panos by Miria Matembe, member of Ugandan parliament, chairperson of Action for Development (Acfode), Uganda, August 1990.

41. Philip Meredith, "MEXFAM's youth and male involvement programmes", IPPF, June 1990.

42. Interview with Professor Constance Wofsy, co-director AIDS activities, San Francisco General Hospital, San Francisco, June 1990.

43. Interview with Marie St Cyr, executive director, Women's Action Resource Network (WARN), New York, June 1990.

44. See reference 21.

45. Hilary Standing and Mere Kisekka, "Sexual behaviour in sub-Saharan Africa: a review and annotated bibliography", School of African and Asian Studies, University of Sussex, UK and Department of Sociology, Ahmadu Bello University, Nigeria, prepared for the Overseas Development Administration (ODA), UK, April 1989.

46. See reference 21.

47. E. Williams and others, "An AIDS intervention program in the Cross River state of Nigeria", paper presented at the Second SWAA Workshop, Lagos, May 1990.

48. J. Mull and V. Lopez, "The Missing Link: the cultural connection in the failure of prostitutes to require clients to use condoms despite a health education campaign", *Abstracts of the First International Symposium on education and information about AIDS*, Ixtapa, Mexico, October 1988, P2-71,

49. See reference 21.

50. D. Worth, "Sexual decision-making and AIDS: why condom promotion among vulnerable women is likely to fail", *Studies in Family Planning*, Nov/Dec 1989, Vol 20, No 6, pp297-307.

51. "Women and AIDS in Africa: issues old and new", paper presented by the Society for Women and AIDS in Africa (SWAA), at the 1989 Annual Meeting of the African Studies Association, Atlanta, USA, November 1989.

52. See reference 42.

53. Report for Panos by Kathe Karlson, Upper Manhattan Task Force on AIDS, New York, September 1989.

54. Edwige Bienvenu-Ba and others, "Experience de la mise sur pied d'un programme de réinsertion et de reconversion d'une population presentant un haut risque de contamination à HIV à Kaolack (Senegal), paper presented at the SWAA 1990 Workshop, Lagos, May 1990.